STOP OVEREATING

EVERYTHING YOU SHOULD KNOW TO END

BINGE EATING AND IMPROVE

RELATIONSHIP WITH FOOD

JESSICA LANE

Table of Contents

Introduction

A lot of people judge the obese and the overweight as being lazy and having weak self-control. In reality, very few people understand that binge eating is a symptom of a bigger issue. People that tell a person with a binge eating disorder to just stop eating usually don't have much idea about this very serious condition. The sad thing about binge eating disorder or compulsive eating is that the person is not even hungry. It just shows that something is really wrong.

Unfortunately, not all that have a binge eating disorder or those that have a tendency to do compulsive eating get help and treatment for their condition. They will often feel embarrassed by their appearance and they won't want to discuss their eating habits with anyone. As a result, they go through life living a vicious cycle of eating huge amounts of food for comfort, feeling guilt and self-loathing, falling into depression, and turning back to food in order to feel better again.

If you are eating compulsively and would like to stop, it's time to evaluate your life. Continuing with your destructive eating habits can only lead to more sadness and health problems. Do some self-searching and identify what you are really hungry for and feed that hunger. Put down your fork and explore your opportunities. Take control of your life right now and stop letting your mouth and your stomach lead you. Get help from people that care about you and talk to a therapist if necessary. Obtain all the help that you need in order to take back control of yourself and live the life you deserve.

There are different causes of overeating, including psychological, emotional, chemical, and physiological. There is no good reason to eat until you are uncomfortable. While nearly everyone overeats once in a while, overeating regularly and feeling unable to stop even when you are full can be a problem.

If left unchecked, overeating habits can often result in major health issues. It is important to make a commitment to control your eating habit. Gain control of your urges to overeat and stop this bad behavior before it ruins your health and well-being. Use these simple steps to help you stop overeating once and for all.

As you embark on the journey to overcome overeating, it is important to point out that the journey will not be easy. You will have moments when you relapse, overeat, and feel bad about yourself and even want to binge even the more. However, you need to pick yourself up, learn from your mistakes, and implement effective guidelines that will help you stay on track. You will also have moments when you think that it is too hard and you just want to give up. During such times, remember how far you have come and get the motivation to move on by looking at all the benefits you start to benefit. It is also important that you get some form of support, as it is very hard to overcome any addiction without any help. Your family and friends, as well as online forums, can be a source of great support.

Chapter 1: Overeating

What is overeating?

Overeating is a disorder involving food and Eating uncontrollably, resulting in undesirable weight gain or obesity. Overeating controls a lot of lifestyles and threatens to develop into a jolt unless people who have the disorder learn how to comprehend it and take action to obliterate it. Additionally, disordered eating involves eating a lot of meals when a person isn't hungry.

It frequently entails eating large amounts in a brief time, called binge eating or eating during the day and never stopping. It may affect both women and men, and it is not just obese with men and women who suffer.

Eating disorders often start because people lose control of their eating habits, which is something everyone does in their lives from time to time. One of the most common times people overeat is during holidays, especially Thanksgiving. How many times have you thought to yourself that you were going to eat as much as you can before sitting down to a Thanksgiving meal?

Other times, people overeat when they go out to restaurants because they feel like they have to eat everything on their plates. Another way people overeat is by skipping meals to "save room" for a later meal. This tends to happen when people know they are going to a place where a lot of food will be served. However, this can cause overeating because we start to feel that we're hungrier because of our missed meal. So, once we sit down to eat, we tend to overeat because we're eating fast, and we feel that because we "saved room," we can eat more than we usually would. In reality, this is a form of overeating because skipping a meal makes your metabolism slow down.

Another common cause of overeating is how fast many people eat. According to researchers, it takes twenty minutes for your stomach to get the signal from your brain to let you know that it's full. Because we eat so fast, our brain and stomach are unable to keep up with us, which means we don't get this signal until after we've been full some time.

Overeating doesn't become a huge problem until people do it twice or more a week for about six months. When this occurs, you've turned your overeating into binge eating.

When Overeating Turns into Binge Eating

Other than the time frame, there are many different ways to tell when overeating turns into binge eating. One of the biggest ways is by paying attention to your emotions. People who overeat occasionally don't tend to have any emotions associated with their overeating. The closest thing many come to making reference to bring emotions into overeating is when people state something like "I shouldn't have eaten so much" or "I can't believe I ate all that!" To people who just overeat occasionally, they overeat, might talk about how they overate, and then don't think about it again.

This isn't the case for someone who binge eats. When a person binge eats, they feel emotions before, during, and after their binge-eating episode. Not only do people who binge eat tend to feel embarrassed, but they also feel ashamed, mad, sad, or frustrated that they allowed themselves to take part in another binge-eating episode. They often feel isolated because they believe they're suffering alone. Many also feel that if they talk to someone about their binge eating or go for help, they will be judged or excluded from family and friends. They hold a lot of fear internally, which only contributes to their binge eating. For many, they haven't even realized they have an eating disorder.

Overeating versus Binge Eating

Before we get too far into overeating and its causes, I first want to explain the difference between binge eating and overeating. Because binge eating has often been described as when a person overeats, people have started to believe that they are nearly the same thing or confuse the terms. But binge eating and overeating are two different terms and conditions.

Overeating is what people tend to do occasionally more than weekly. For example, during holidays, social events, and parties. There are several differences between binge eating and overeating. First, to be considered a binge eater, you need to overeat at least twice a week for at least six months. Other than the time frame, binge eaters become upset over the amount they've eaten. If you overeat and you don't feel emotional about your overeating, then you won't be classified as a binge eater by a professional. Another difference with a binge eater is they eat from emotional cues. They don't feel the cue from their body on being full or hungry. They eat because of their emotions. Finally, binge eaters avoid eating in public places, which includes in front of family and friends. For them, eating should be done in a private setting where they are allowed to eat alone.

Why Millennials Overeat

Nearly everyone overeats at one time or another, but experts believe that at least 75 percent of people overeat due to boredom or other reasons and not because of hunger.[1] There are a variety of reasons why people overeat. Other than the typical holidays and social outings, people can also overeat because they are bored, or they're watching a movie or television show. Many people tend to overeat because they are eating in a mindless way. Meaning, they aren't thinking about how much they are eating. Mindless eating often happens when people are focusing on other things, such as on their phone or in front of the television, instead of focusing on the food in front of them. Because their focus is elsewhere, they don't pay attention to the cues from their stomach telling them they're full.

People might also overeat now and then because they're on vacation. When people are on vacation, they want to try as many different foods as possible. Emotions also play a role in overeating. For example, if you've had a bad day at work, you might eat more than your regular portion because you feel it'll make you feel better. Others tend to overeat for a period of time when they stop smoking because their food tastes better than it used to. Women tend to overeat during their menstrual cycle. Another reason people eat is because they had to clean off their plates as children.

Why Millennials Binge Eat

Just as there are many reasons people overeat, there are dozens of reasons people binge eat. No one has been able to pinpoint direct reasons to why people binge eat. In fact, I'm not going to be able to cover all the reasons because let's be honest, it's different for so many people. We're all our own person, and with this, comes our own problems and our own ways to deal with them. However, I am going to discuss several of the most common reasons people binge eat.

Emotional Reasons

Many millennials cite emotional reasons for why they became a binge eater. Because of various situations they were going through or went through in their lives, they turned to food. For them, food became their comfort, which it does for everyone now and then. How many times have you had a bad day and decided to stop at the store and grab a bag of chips or candy or went through a fast food drive-through for supper? If so, you're not alone. In fact, this is done daily by people all over. Psychologically, food is often a comfort for most people because it satisfies us, and we are looking for any type of satisfaction in order to help us get through our bad day or help us cope with our situation.

The emotions people deal with that often lead them to binge eat are negative emotions, such as anger, frustration, loneliness, and sadness. While it's not impossible, it's more uncommon for people to binge eat when they're feeling positive emotions, such as happiness or pride. People are more likely to engage in overeating other than binge eating because they feel positive emotions.

Psychological

Internal psychological struggles, such as low self-esteem and depression, have a strong correlation to binge eating. This is also known to go both ways. People who are depressed can start to binge eat, and people who binge eat can become depressed. Because this is so common, it's been hard for researchers to figure out which one, either binge eating or depression, is more of the cause and which is more of the effect.

Through research, scientists have been able to conclude that at least half the people who binge eat are depressed. They also don't have to show signs of depression at that time as they could have a history of depression, which most likely means the binge eating started with a depressive episode.

Dr. Cynthia Bulik, a professor of eating disorders from the University of North Carolina at Chapel Hill, states that studies show that you can be born with risks for both depression and binge eating.

Stress

Along with emotion, many millennials cite stress as one of the reasons they started to binge eat. Like with emotions, comfort food helped them cope with the stress they felt in their daily life. This stress could come from many sources, but for many, it came from their jobs, class schedule, financial problems, and family life.

Any generation that came before millennials can't deny that starting a career, struggling with finances, and raising a family aren't a struggle from time to time. However, many people from these generations also feel that struggles have become worse since they started their own families and careers. One of the biggest reasons for this is because of inflation. Everything from purchasing a home to buying groceries has increased dramatically over the years. Unfortunately, minimum wage and the typical hourly wage business owners pay haven't increased as dramatically. Because of this, financial problems among millennials have worsened, which causes more stress in their daily lives.

Another major stress component that has increased since the previous generations are mixing career and family. In order for a millennial couple to live paycheck to paycheck, both have to work full-time jobs. When you mix this in with the fact that they are also raising families, it becomes more stressful. Previously, one spouse, which was usually the wife, stayed home to take care of the house and family. But this isn't possible for the majority of millennial couples, and because of this, they are struggling with higher levels of stress, which increases a couple's disagreements. In response, couples get more stressed and unhappy because of their disagreements.

Genetics

For years, researchers studied if there was a link between binge eating and genetics. A few years ago, Dr. Camron Bryant and his colleagues from Boston University School of Medicine finally made a breakthrough and discovered that the gene CYFIP2 was associated with binge eating. This meant that if the parent suffered from binge eating, his or her child held a higher risk for developing binge eating disorder over children whose parents never suffered from binge eating. Researchers identified the gene cytoplasmic FMR1-interacting protein 2 or CYFIP2 through gene validation and mapping. Their research concluded that this gene was a risk factor for binge eating.

Due to these findings, Bryant believes that the psychiatric field can work to improve their therapies surrounding binge eating and other eating disorders. Bryant stated that he believes by doing this, they will be able to not only more efficiently help people but also save more lives.

It Just Happened

Sometimes there are no real underlying reasons for why you became a binge eater. It simply just happened. For many people, this is more real than others might think. It can easily happen when you start to make a habit out of overeating. Before you realize it, your overeating has turned into binge eating. At this point, the only thing people can do is hope that they can realize their binge eating habits before it's too late.

Of course, there are many other reasons that people binge eat, and no one's reasoning is wrong. If you know why you tend to overeat or binge eat, don't be embarrassed or feel that the reason isn't like anyone else's reasoning, or you shouldn't let the problem or emotions you have make you binge eat. In order to overcome binge eating, you need to accept the reason and find ways to overcome overeating, whether it's through the pages of this book or another means. You can overcome overeating, binge eating, or any eating disorder you're currently facing.

There are many tricks which can help you figure out your stomach's cues to tell you that you're full so you don't overeat. The trick to quit eating when you're really full is to know how to eat. For instance, you want to eat slowly. The slower you eat, the more likely you are to catch that feeling of fullness when you've hit your mark. In a fast-paced world, we're used to eating quickly, but this is going to make up overeat because our system moves slower than we do when we're eating. Another trick is to portion out your meals. This means that you take the time to measure out the food you'll be eating.

A final trick, one which I encourage you to try, is to notice how your stomach feels when you feel hungry. Once you feel this sensation, drink a glass of water and then pay attention to how your stomach feels. This will help you better understand the feeling your stomach gives when you're reaching your level of fullness.

Chapter 2: Body Focus

What Can Your Body Do?

You need to learn how to listen to your body. There is a difference between emotional and physical hunger. Your body is only capable of consuming so much of anything, pushing it further than it can take will cause numerous problems.

Don't punish yourself and your body, for your bad eating habits. Focus on what you can, and cannot do. When changing your habits, food, interests and lifestyle, your body will adapt to the changes, so learn to listen to what it is telling you.

If your stomach is not growling, you may only be experiencing a craving. Allow it to pass, get busy doing other things that you have added to your 'keep busy list'.

Focus each activity on your abilities, and only do what you can. Do not push your body past its own abilities, this could end up doing more harm to your body, than good.

Be proud of your accomplishments, however small they may be. In time you will grow. Your capabilities will become more prominent, and you will see an internal strength come to light. One you never even knew was there.

Actions

Go through the actions, not only to get things done, but with focus. Focus on everything you do, consider before acting and make sure you are doing only what you can. Talk to yourself, ask yourself before going forward, consider the options and weigh them up against each other.

We all have habits and these need to change. Bad habits need to be replaced with good ones. Consider things before just falling head first into something that may cause mental, or physical strain.

Make a list of things to do, and actions to take when the need to eat arises. Write down your goals for each week. These can include exercises, fun activities, chats with friends or family, or reading, writing and spending time with your pets, or children playing games.

Make all of these your new habits, do it on a daily and weekly basis.

Chapter 3: Self-Analysis

Self-Esteem

You need to sit down, and be completely honest with yourself. You can lie to others, but when you start lying to yourself, you may have bigger problems surfacing.

People with binge disorder usually suffer from low self-esteem, and may also have low self-respect. You need to realize, you are unique, you are special, and only you can change the way you see yourself.

This will not be easy, and it will surely be quite a rocky road to travel, nonetheless, you can achieve it. Look at yourself in the mirror every morning, and compliment yourself on your looks.

When you do something, and you do it well or get praised for it, accept it and also praise yourself. Build up your self-esteem over time and you will succeed. Honesty will take you far, so trust yourself and those closest to you.

Give yourself a lift, and motivate yourself by telling yourself the good, positive things you have in life. Do this in the mornings, and evening before going to bed.

No-One Is Perfect

Don't try to be perfect, no-one is, no-one! Not even the movie actors, models or stars are perfect. We all have flaws, some have just learned how to hide theirs better than others. So, stop trying!

Setting too high, or unrealistic goals may lead to mental issues developing over time. This is due to not being able to reach them these goals. We are each made unique, we experience life different, and our experiences change the way we perceive things. Consequently, no one is perfect, or even the same as another, not even identical twins.

So, stop trying to be whom, or what you are not. Accept yourself and your unique qualities.

Perfectionists are also prone to become consumed by binge eating. They believe their health foods, their ways to be correct, and this is not always the case. They can become very unhappy people, always seeking better, cleaner and more efficient ways to live. This can lead to depression, anxiety and cause great stress.

Once binge eating takes a hold on you, it is harder to let go, than it is preventing it in the first place. Voltaire had a quote that sums it up exceptionally well, "Perfect is the enemy of good." This says it all, so get rid of any thoughts you may hold of perfection, there is no such thing in life.

Chapter 4: Therapy Methods

Group Therapy

Binge eating disorder is much like any other addiction. And at some point or the other, you are going to need support. Group therapy is ideal for everyone struggling with this disease. As you can see there are others out there with the same problems, you are not alone. Not everyone has the same reasons for it, or look the same, or even react the same to situations, but you are not alone, and this is comforting.

Breaking this pattern is not easy, and sometlmes you may even slip up. That is why it is so extremely important to have a support group. You can join one if there is one close to you, ask your therapist and find out about groups you could join in your area. Or you can make your own one, include supportive family members and friends, and/or even your therapist.

Sharing your experiences, what goes through your mind and how it feels, can help you as well as others understand, but may also aid you in realizing when it happens. If you feel a binge attack coming on call someone, talk it out and allow others to help you move on.

Group therapy includes discussions on healthy eating patterns, and how to cope with urges, in addition to making new friends. Getting to know people who are like you, with a common goal in life.

Hypnosis

Hypnosis can be a strong form of treatment, if done by a professional. With hypnosis, habits can be suggestively altered over time. You can be motivated to stop habits that are ruining your life, and new good habits can begin to form. This treatment however, needs to be done by a trained professional.

It will also take time, as it is not a question of having one session, and now all problems are solved. Hypnosis addresses the underlying issue, the cause of your binge eating. With hypnosis the triggers that bring on your binge eating sessions are targeted, the emotions that cause one to react to situations, and feelings by eating.

What can be achieved with hypnosis? Hypnosis assists in the replacement of your emotional response to the triggers that are causing you to binge. With hypnosis your mind is allowed to form a different response to the things that usually set you off. You will be more aware, and will be able to make a sensible choice when presented with a trigger.

The suggested length of treatment may be anything from three weeks, to three months. This will mostly depend on your binge habits, as well as the therapist treating you.

Chapter 5: You have all the willpower you need

One of the cruelest lies told to us is that overweight people are heavy because they lack willpower.

It only takes the most casual observation to realize the falsity of this, however, this negative judgment is built into the very fabric of our society. We are taught to feel ashamed of ourselves if our bodies are more than svelte; ashamed at our lack of willpower.

There's a real wickedness here.

It starts in the schoolyard, if not sooner, and is encouraged by judgmental and sadistic adults who project their own inadequacies onto innocent children.

And there is hypocrisy to this judgment too which is not at first apparent but becomes so on reflection: it is far easier to lose five or ten pounds than fifty or a hundred, but how many people who look down on the overweight or obese are themselves over their ideal weight?

A so-called average person with a "few pounds" to lose criticizing a morbidly obese person is analogous to someone who can't walk a block criticizing a marathon runner for running slowly!

Those fortunate enough to live under modern conditions, including a modern diet and a largely sedentary lifestyle, without experiencing much difficulty in controlling their weight are lucky rather than virtuous.

Genetics are the first and chief determinant of weight. But genetic expression is influenced by environment. The hormones which wash over the fetus in the womb affect how the developing baby's genes will express. This is what accounts for the differences between identical twins.

Obesity was unknown among the indigenous inhabitants of North America. Once the food supply changed for them obesity — and related problems such as diabetes — soared. They have the same genes they had before they encountered Europeans, but those genes now express very differently.

And you can observe a similar result in the ancestors of those very Europeans — us.

One need only look at pictures of North Americans from the 70s to see how slender people were back then in comparison to today.

This is due to the change in our food supply rather than changes in our activity level. People obsess about fitness now far more than they did in the 70's. Back then it was a rare thing to go to a gym; now it's a rare thing for a hotel or condominium complex not to have at least a fitness room.

We are as a society much heavier than formerly. This is not the result of the diminishment of our collective willpower. We subject ourselves voluntarily to stricter regimens of diet and exercise that any of our ancestors — including those of even a few decades ago — ever did.

Our earliest ancestors, of course, ate as much as they could, and rested at every opportunity. All organisms do. It's how they survive in a competitive world of scarcity.

But the people living back in the 70's weren't hunters and gatherers. They were pretty much like us (indeed you may be one of them) so why were they so much slimmer?

We've mentioned changes in the food supply, but while that may have started the ball rolling something more insidious has kept it going and even caused it to pick up speed.

How many diets have you been on?

Most people reading this book have been on more diets than they can count. Some of these diets have been strict, or even severe — think Master cleanse — and all of them have been completely contrary to our natural impulse which is to eat to satiety and beyond whenever food is available.

It takes a Herculean effort to restrict our caloric intake voluntarily when food is available. And yet you have done this, exactly this, and not just for a day or two but for protracted periods and very likely repeatedly.

You've demonstrated prodigious willpower in overcoming millennia of evolutionary programming, and you've done so time and time again.

Chances are, notwithstanding your repeated displays of willpower, that your weight has continued to increase over time. This weight-gain may be partly due to age and hormonal changes.

But it is also due to the well-known yo-yo effect of dieting where you lost ten pounds and gained back fifteen as a result of changes to your body composition — essentially, replacing muscle with fat even as weight loss is occurring— and as a consequence of the rebound eating which occurs after a period of deprivation.

Yes, this is where your willpower has gotten you: right in the middle of a vicious circle where you grow larger and more desperate each passing year.

You not only have more willpower than you need — you have more willpower than is good for you.

Willpower is necessary to achieve many goals. It will help you in completing your education, in furthering your career, and with fitness, financial, and spiritual goals, but it's a positive hindrance to your efforts to achieve and sustain your weight loss goals.

Using willpower to attempt to control your eating puts you at risk of, not just the vicious circle described above, but also of developing eating disorders.

Eating disorders, such as bulimia and anorexia nervosa, are beyond the scope of this book. If you have symptoms of either, you should immediately consult your physician. Both can have serious health consequences and can even be fatal.

The force you exert through willpower is met by an equal and opposing force. The harder you try to force yourself to abstain from food, the harder your survival instincts push back and urge you to eat. The more willpower you employ, the more opposition you create.

Studies have shown that chronic dieters have an elevation of the hormone in the amygdala which causes the negative emotional effect that drives overeating. The changes in their brains are similar to the changes observed in the brains of alcoholics and drug addicts and the anxiety and compulsion to overeat are similar to the anxiety and compulsion alcoholics and drug addicts experience to consume alcohol and drugs.

This is the legacy of using willpower to repeatedly override the survival drive to eat of the amygdala to eat when stressed and produces the same vicious cycle experienced by chronic abuse of alcohol and drugs.

Stress leads to negative emotions which turn on the survival drive to overeat which, when suppressed through willpower, become stronger until overeating occurs changing the brain so that the urge to consume food becomes as strong as an alcoholic's urge to consume alcohol or a drug addict's urge to consume drugs.

The more you use your willpower to diet, and the stricter your diets have been, the more you have exposed yourself to the operation of your survival drives which are programmed to ensure your survival by driving you to consume food.

When you use your willpower to restrict your caloric intake, this has the same effect on your lower brain as actual starvation. Indeed, from the standpoint of your lower brain, there is no difference between voluntarily ceasing to eat, and not eating because no food is available.

Disabuse yourself of the notion that you lack willpower. And also disabuse yourself of the idea that you need willpower to achieve your weight loss goals or to control your eating. Nothing could be further from the truth.

Emotional eating is not a disorder of the will, nor is it a lack of self-discipline, or lack of self-control. Instead, emotional eating is caused by and exacerbated by using your willpower to mimic the effect of starvation thus triggering your survival drives which urge you to eat.

The stronger your willpower, the stronger the urges to eat which come from your lower, ancient brain.

And not only does it works better, it can actually be enjoyable!

Your Ancient Brain

You and your amygdala

When we start a diet, we have the best of intentions.

We've done our research, have decided on a diet plan that we believe will work for us — this time for sure! — and convinced ourselves that we intend to stick to it.

And often we do, for day or two, or a week or two, and then the inevitable happens: we succumb to the temptation of delicious food and eat things that we've determined not to, or in larger quantities than we ought, or both.

The stricter the diet, the more likely we are to obsess about food and the worse our binge is likely to be when we finally break down and start eating.

It's as though a part of us is in diametric opposition to our better judgment. A part so strong, and incessant, that we eventually yield to its urgings.

It can't be us, can it? How can we be so at war with ourselves?

We aren't at war with ourselves. We are at war with our lower, or primitive, brain.

This ancient brain is the seat of our survival instincts. It is often called the old brain, or reptilian brain, and it has a limited repertoire of responses to stimuli which are hardwired.

It is concerned with basic survival and procreation. It doesn't have the capacity to plan or think of the future. Instead, it responds in simple preprogrammed ways.

When we experience the "fight or flight" response to a threat, it's our reptilian brain that has responded, and it can act much quicker than we can reason. We can be aroused sexually without any conscious input. It is our reptilian brain that drives us to eat when food is available.

Our neocortex, the rational part of our brain that makes us human and makes us decide to do things like attempt to reduce our weight, is a relatively recent addition. Our ancestors survived for countless millennia without it.

And our ancestors survived just fine. That's because the lower brain that they relied on worked perfectly to ensure their survival.

They were driven to eat when food was available, to flee or fight to defend themselves and to procreate, and thus pass on their genes. We are the end product.

So we should be grateful to the survival brain for getting us to the stage where we can make choices rather than operate by simple instinct.

It's hard to feel grateful, however, when our survival brain is importuning us to eat foods that are harming our health.

The survival brain works on the principle that "if it feels good do it." No thinking is required. It drives us to eat, have sex, and even to be lazy and conserve our energy when neither is available.

Our survival brain isn't trying to harm us when it urges us to eat or even overeat. It is trying to keep us alive.

We are told to be mindful when we are eating so that we can be aware when we are full, and stop eating.

This is good advice in dealing with our survival brain — which is never full when ample delicious food is available — and can work reasonably well when things are going smoothly in our lives.

Being mindful while we were eating means that our cerebral cortex is engaged which enables us to make rational decisions about our food intake.

The failure to be mindful and aware while eating can lead to us "wolfing" our food down — and it's no accident that we refer to it as "wolfing;" our language recognizes that it is the lower or animal part of our brain which engages in this behavior — and eating far more than we intend to.

The problem arises when we are unable to be mindful. This is when emotional eating kicks in. It's difficult to be mindful and calmly aware of your eating when you are upset, stressed, angry, lonely or feeling unloved.

When things are not going smoothly in our lives, the need for the comfort that food can provide is too great for us to resist the importunings of our survival brain. Sooner or later we give in to its relentless urgings and indulge in forbidden food.

Our survival brain is ancient and implacable.

We cannot fight it on its terms. It is far too patient, relentless and indefatigable for us to hope to beat it head on.

But it does have one profound disadvantage: it is completely unable to take action on its own.

Your survival brain can urge you to eat. It can tempt you with thoughts of delicious food. It can assault your consciousness with endless imagery of the wonderful culinary options readily available to you. It can remind you yet again how empty your tummy is.

But it cannot open the refrigerator door. It cannot lift a single morsel of food to your lips.

Your survival brain is powerless to take any action contrary to your conscious will, or even to take any action at all.

It is in thrall to your cerebral cortex. It can't fix itself dinner; it is wholly dependent on you.

Although it can exert tremendous influence over you, it has no power to compel you to act.

And therein lies the key to ensuring dominance over it: you must recognize its urgings for what they are; they are not you but rather your survival instincts.

Do not think of it as an adversary but rather as an ally, a powerful force that can be used for good or ill.

There is no need to demonize it or label it in a pejorative way any more than you would do that to an animal in your care.

We don't describe a begging dog as being wayward or wrongheaded, just greedy. You don't give the dog more treats than are good for him, but you don't judge him.

You can deal with your survival brain in the same way.

In fact, it's helpful to think of your survival brain in a friendly, even indulgent, way like the way you would think of a pet. Your survival brain is acting out of instinct and has no choice concerning the nature of its desires.

Like a pet, your survival brain lives in the now. It has no concept of the future; neither does it dwell in the past. It lives in the present, and in the present tasty food is always good. It is not rational; it precedes reason.

You, on the other hand, are able to make rational choices. You can appreciate the future consequences of the choices you make in the moment. And you are the one in control.

The neocortex or modern brain has dominion over the primitive brain in the same manner that humans have dominion over the animal kingdom.

So you can see that, as powerful as the primitive brain is, it has no ability to act independently of your modern rational brain.

You, that is to say, your neocortex, is in complete control at all times. The only way that your survival brain can gain the upper hand, and cause you to eat more than you wish to, or choose foods which you wish to avoid, is if you let it.

You'll soon learn how to stop it in its tracks, and later how to train it much as you might train a pet.

But first, we'll solve a puzzle that has doubtless tormented you over the years more cruelly than even the most challenging crossword ever could: why do you eat when you're not hungry?

Chapter 6: Methods and Treatments to Overcome Food Addiction

In this chapter, we will learn all about the different methods that professionals use to treat Binge Eating Disorder. We will find out how each method differs from one another, what their core philosophies are, and how they can each effectively treat BED in their own way.

Mindfulness Meditation

You might feel completely powerless whenever your cravings hit, but you actually have more control over your binge eating than you might realize. A simple act of taking five minutes' break before giving in to your urges helps you practice mindfulness. Before you dig into a particularly sinful treat, pause and reflect on what you are about to do. Put off reaching for that tub of ice cream for about five minutes, and tell yourself to wait.

During this quick moment of silence, allow yourself the opportunity of reflecting on your emotions. How will this food make you feel? Why exactly do you need this food? What is happening inside your deepest emotions, and what kind of inner turmoil are you experiencing right now? Meditating on why you want to eat what you want to eat helps you understand your craving, making you more and more mindful of what you consume.

With this meditation comes acceptance of your deepest feelings, both good and bad. Cut yourself some slack by letting yourself feel these emotions, even if they are not all positive. While these unpleasant feelings may be overwhelmingly uncomfortable at first, you will eventually learn not to fear these negative energies and instead learn to understand and accept them. This kind of connection with your negative feelings lets you handle your stress more effectively, leading to better emotional coping mechanisms. Now, isn't that an incredible feat to accomplish in just five minutes?

Dialectical Behavioral Therapy

What Is Dialectical Behavior Therapy? Dialectical Behavior Therapy (DBT) provides therapy on four focused areas in order to help clients manage their negative emotions. These therapeutic skills provided assist patients with decreasing conflict in their relationships, thereby improving how they interact socially with others.

There are four key areas in Dialectical Behavior Therapy. This focuses on an individual's power to accept what is currently in the moment. The second area is distress tolerance, which helps improve a person's ability to tolerate negative emotions. This is focused on keeping a patient from trying to escape his or her negative emotions.

The third is emotion regulation. This helps patients manage their intense emotions so as not to let these disrupt his or her life. And finally, the fourth is interpersonal effectiveness. This teaches patients various techniques to help an individual communicate properly with others, all in the context of maintaining assertiveness and self-respect. This allows the person to have stronger relationships with others in the long run.

Initially, DBT was developed in the 1980s by Marsha Linehan, Ph.D. in order to help treat borderline personality disorder. This cognitive-behavioral treatment has successfully helped people who have trouble managing negative emotions, causing uncontrollable and intense negative emotions whenever a person interacts with others. It doesn't matter if it's a romantic partner, a family member, or a friend—those who suffer from the condition are often still unable to interact well with them, experiencing extreme difficulty in their relationships.

Now, DBT is also being used successfully to treat various disorders like binge eating, post-traumatic stress disorder, bipolar disorder, substance abuse, bulimia, and depression. It is especially effective for people who need help in regulating their emotions and in tolerating extreme distress and other intense negative emotions. DBT allows a person to take back his life by being present in the now, being mindful of others, and being able to communicate and interact well with society.

With individual therapy sessions of DBT, a patient is assured that all of his therapeutic needs are met by a one-on-one trained therapist. The sessions will help the patient apply the skills learned in DBT in his day-to-day life, keep him motivated, and help him overcome obstacles and various struggles that he may face during the treatment.

With group therapy sessions, participants can learn and apply their skills with others in the group. Everyone is encouraged to speak up and share their own personal experiences, allowing them to get involved in various exercises to provide mutual support for everyone. Professional therapists teach skills and assign homework for all participants, which includes practicing mindfulness and the likes. These sessions can go on weekly for about half a year, and each session can last for about two hours.

In essence, DBT is characterized by trying to balance out opposites. From the name itself, dialectics are important—the therapist makes sure that the patient is able to balance out two complete opposites without resorting to a black-and-white approach to social situations. At the heart of DBT is not an all-or-nothing way of thinking but one that promotes acceptance and positive change.

For instance, when applied to BED, DBT helps by finding a middle ground for two extremes. One opposite here is following a diet plan strictly and absolutely, allowing no room for any kind of slip-up whatsoever. The other opposite is being more relaxed when it comes to adhering to your abstinence. This polar opposite supports the fact that following your meal plan is just utterly impossible.

How, then, can DBT help find a synthesis between the two? This method teaches patients that there should be a balance between the two extremes. You are going to lapse from your strict diet plan at some point, and that's okay. You really can't plan for total and complete adherence. What matters is that you can cope with these lapses in a healthy way. DBT teaches patients to regulate their emotions. Proper distress tolerance skills are developed so that a person suffering from BED can overcome the hurdle of giving in to a food craving and moving on to prevent spiralling down toward another harmful eating behavior and making things worse.

As such, it is extremely important to find the right therapist for you. A good Dialectical Behavior Therapist must also learn to practice the skills learned as well, able to understand the patient's experiences and behaviors. A therapist must be professionally certified and qualified to apply basic behavior therapy as well as the proper DBT strategies. Above all, it's crucial to find a therapist that you are comfortable with.

Cognitive Behavioral Therapy

What is Cognitive Behavioral Therapy? CBT helps modify emotions, thoughts, and behaviors that are dysfunctional in order to increase a person's overall happiness. The method focuses on looking for solutions to underlying problems not through traditional Freudian psychoanalysis but through encouraging to change their destructive behaviors and face their distorted patterns of cognition. It doesn't try to delve deep into a person's childhood wounds to try to pinpoint root causes of problems, but rather, it aims to help identify which harmful thoughts distort a person's depiction of reality. If these negative thoughts are found to be inaccurate, then CBT develops strategies to help a person challenge these notions and ultimately overcome them.

Of course, this isn't to say that the patient's past is irrelevant. Trained CBT therapists must also consider the patient's history and previous experiences, as these help shape who we are today. How we think greatly influences how we act, and CBT helps to understand the psychological learning history of the patient in order to arrive at a thorough assessment for treatment.

CBT believes firmly that a person's perceptions greatly influence his or her behavior. If you're feeling down in the dumps, it could only be due to your distorted perception of what's actually real. With this method, people of all ages can be treated, including those suffering from major depressive disorder, post-traumatic stress disorder, anxiety disorders, obsessive-compulsive disorders, and, of course, Binge Eating Disorder.

In the Behavioral Phase of CBT, the therapist addresses negative emotions and helps minimize these behaviors such as episodic overeating related to shame. The therapist educates the patient on balanced eating and proper meal planning, then, he or she helps come up with strategies to manage the emotions that lead to the binge. This includes skills on thought stopping, distracting one's self, and prolonging urges.

In the Cognitive Phase, patients are taught how to challenge the way they think. Cognitive Restructuring also involves teaching patients how to identify the unhealthy thoughts that lead them astray from the road to BED recovery. The therapist helps a person conquer their distorted thoughts on their body image and self-worth. They tackle unrealistic expectations on beauty and perfection, slowly enabling a patient to gain insight on how to be more hopeful and embrace changing for the better.

Interpersonal Psychotherapy

What is Interpersonal Psychotherapy? IPT helps treat mood disorders by helping improve a patient's relationships and social interactions in order to decrease overall stress. This evidence-based approach also focuses on four key areas. First, interpersonal deficits are assessed to see if the person is suffering from any kind of social isolation or is involved in an unfulfilling relationship with someone. Second, IPT helps people deal with any unresolved grief, whether it involves a past or recent death. Third, patients are encouraged to learn how to handle unpleasant transitions in life, which includes moving, retirement, or even divorce. The fourth and final area deals with conflicts between expectations from loved ones and acquaintances. Aside from treating BED, IPT can also be used to treat major depressive disorder, perinatal depression, alcohol addiction, substance addiction, dysthymia, and bipolar disorder.

What makes IPT different from other approaches is that it analyzes current relationships rather than previous ones. It focuses on internal conflicts, and can be less directive than other cognitive behavioral methods. It does, however, also have both one-on-one and group therapy sessions. Treatment includes assignments, ongoing assessments, and therapist interviews. As the treatment continuously progresses, and after depressive symptoms have been examined, both therapist and patient work together to develop treatment strategies that target a person's particular problem areas. Group sessions have interpersonal dynamics that provide opportunities and a safe environment for all patients to practice their learned skills with a strong, supportive community.

Practitioners of IPT believe that depression stems from a change in a person's social environment. Your licensed therapist should be able to help you determine your interpersonal issues, as well as provide you with support on analyzing communication skills and listening to you supportively.

In this chapter, we learned that practicing mindfulness meditation can be as simple as taking a break for five minutes to pause for a while before taking action on our impulses. This method helps curb any negative cravings, especially when it comes to BED. We also learned that Dialectical Behavior Therapy can help patients manage their negative emotions better in order to decrease conflicts in their relationships. This, in turn, helps improve a person's social interactions with others.   Cognitive Behavioral Therapy, on the other hand, focuses on assessing whether or not a person's thoughts and perceptions are distorted. It aims to correct these negative perceptions to improve a person's behavior.   Finally,   Interpersonal Psychotherapy focuses on improving a person's overall quality of life by diagnosing current relationships to decrease overall stress.

Chapter 7: Food Cravings

Another reason why following the latest detox fad won't help you create lasting change is cravings. Restrictive dieting tends to cause even stronger cravings in people, for their favorite unhealthy snacks. Ask any person out there what type of food they typically crave, and chances are, they will have a couple of items that automatically come to mind. This is because cravings happen as a result of our habits.

It's Natural and Okay to Crave Foods:
The first key thing to realize now is that it is okay to have food cravings. That's right; any time you beat yourself up for wanting that slice of pie after lunch or wishing desperately for a bacon cheese burger, you're being unnecessarily harsh on yourself. By accepting that cravings are natural and should, in fact, be expected, you are actually helping the craving to dissolve. Think about it, are you less or more prepared for something when you expect it? Telling yourself that cravings are unacceptable just makes you unprepared to handle them when they occur, and far more likely to buckle under the temptation. Consider the following points:

• Everyone has Food Cravings: Studies show that basically all humans, men and women, have experienced cravings for some type of food in the last year. It's nothing to be ashamed of, and it's actually partially to thank for helping us evolve.

• It's all Mental: People who aren't as prone to succumbing to their cravings might tell others that these thoughts are purely mental, and studies show that this is absolutely correct. It is all in your mind! Actually, our pleasure center and memory center in the brain are responsible for these food cravings. Our brains come to associate certain foods with rewards, and this leads us to want more.

Research has proven that dampening the opiate centers of the brain actually dampen cravings for sugary and fatty foods, proving that pleasure has a lot to do with our experience of them.

• Less Stress means Fewer Cravings: One major step you can take to diminish the level of cravings you feel is lessening stress in your life. Although there are physiological explanations behind cravings for food, they are also related to desire and general emotions. We crave foods because they can satisfy needs we have, like getting rid of anxiety or reducing stress. For a lot of us, an episode of stress or anxiety can cause severe and instant cravings.

Carbs heighten our serotonin levels, calming us down quickly. Studies have also suggested that sugar and fat, when combined, produce an effect of calming. San Francisco University researchers found that rats placed into environments of high stress gravitated toward sugary and fatty foods, which resulted in lower stress levels.

Tips to Help you Handle Food Cravings:
Don't allow those pesky cravings to sabotage your efforts and progress. Instead, follow these guidelines to stay on track to becoming your best weight.

• Be Realistic about your Control Levels: Remember that restricting yourself can cause you to slip off track later. This is not to say that always giving into cravings is good, but be realistic about how much you can control yourself once you begin eating chocolate or a salty snack. Are a few chips or M&Ms enough for you? If so, indulging is perfectly okay, every once in awhile.

However, if you tend to have cravings that spiral deeper, and lead you to finish an entire family sized bag of chips or gallon of cookies and cream, it's time to be honest with yourself. Getting a clear picture of what you're dealing with is the only way to adequately handle it. If you know you're susceptible to overdoing it, try only keeping small portions in the house. For example, buy a single serving back of chips, or buy one slice of cake, rather than an entire cake.

- Try for Healthier Options: When possible, try going for lower calorie dishes, whenever you can. You might immediately think that this won't satisfy you as much as what you're used to, but it all depends on how creative you get. Changes are, putting Greek yogurt on top of your meals, instead of sour cream, will satisfy you just as much once you get used to it. Although we are constantly surrounded by temptation and junk food, which is cheap, easy, and instantly attainable most of the time, it's all a matter of habit. Get used to saying no, and you will rarely even notice the donut shop on your way to work.

- Don't Skip Meals or Become Too Hungry between Them: When you skip meals, or pass up eating when you really needed to, it's likelier that you will overindulge when you get the chance. Again, deprivation breeds a form of desperation and you will wish to overcompensate for the lack you just experienced. It sounds slightly counterintuitive, eating to prevent overeating, but staying satisfied throughout the day will help you prevent binges or uncontrollable cravings.

• Write about your Cravings: For those of you who have severe cravings, try writing about them. Record each time throughout your day that you experience a craving, including what you feel before and during the craving, what food you wanted the most, and how much and what you had to eat earlier. You can then review the information later on to look for patterns in certain emotions leading to cravings, or a specific time of day that you are more susceptible.

• Be Smart about your Carb Choices: We have already gone over the fact that we crave foods high in sugar and fat, including highly refined carbs. And we've gone over the fact that stress leads to craving carbs, since they have a calming effect. This means that the smartest method for calming ourselves down, yet providing our bodies with nourishment, is opting for healthier, "smarter" carbs, such as vegetables, fruits, beans, or grains. These will provide your body with the carbs you're craving, in addition to nutritional strength that lasts from minerals, vitamins, and fiber.

Next time you're craving a toasted sandwich with cheese, opt for bread that is whole wheat instead of white, and go for cheese with lower fat. Next time you have a craving for cake, bake one at home and use flour, made of whole wheat instead of white flour, and a healthier sugar substitute. Try using coconut oil instead of butter.

• Nurture Yourself Physically and Mentally: The majority of people need a healthy dose of self-nurturing in order to thrive and improve their lives. Taking care of yourself emotionally and mentally will lead to less unhappiness, anger, and stress in your life, which will mean you won't crave unhealthy foods as often. If you notice that you are tempted to eat junk food constantly, this could be a signal that you're in need of less stress in your life. How to deal with this is up to you, but you could start by getting out in nature more, spending time with loved ones, or even dedicating more of your free time to a hobby.

NLP Techniques to Eliminate Food Cravings

Technique 1: Asking the Right Questions

In order to win when your food cravings strike, you must first learn to recognize the signs of craving. Here are some ways to tell harmful, potentially destructive cravings for actual hunger:

- *Abruptness:* The first way to tell cravings from legitimate hunger is the fact that hunger comes on slowly, while cravings are abrupt. Did you just finish lunch an hour ago, but suddenly feel the need for chocolate cake? This is a craving, not legitimate hunger or the need to eat.

- *Reflect on your Hunger:* Next time you feel hungry, don't mindlessly reach for the potato chips out of habit. Instead, reflect a bit on the sensation. Are you really hungry? Perhaps it's just thirst, since our brains can often mistake this for hunger. Learn to pause your impulses and figure out the nature of your hunger.

- *Choose what you Need, not what you Want:* When you have determined that you are actually hungry, and needing nutrition, figure out what would make you feel best to eat. Does a certain food sound good, and if so, how do you usually feel after eating that food? Try to go for foods that leave you feeling satisfied, not bloated or craving more.

Technique 2: NLP Swish Technique for Eliminating Food Cravings

Humans have a natural instinct to retreat from undesired or unpleasant experienced, and gravitate toward pleasurable behaviors or experiences, in life. The NLP Swish technique uses this instinct for positive results, essentially guiding you into new patterns of feeling, thinking, and ultimately, acting. You could, for instance, pick up an attitude like fear of heights, or a habit like smoking.

• Identifying the Roots: This next section will allow you to identify how your problem with weight gain or excessive eating became an issue in the first place, using the Swish technique. Then you will be asked to find out where and when you would wish to respond or act differently than your old ingrained ways. Let's look at an example. If your problem is late night pizza cravings, and you can attribute much of your weight problems to this behavior, you may be able to recall when this began, and who you were with the first time you started doing this. You may also be able to look back at this memory and figure out what you wish you would have done instead, or how you would have reacted if you had another chance to go back before this pattern became truly ingrained.

• Your Cue Image: The next step will be identifying a mental picture, or cue, of the time that you first began this habit. Most people walk around throughout their days on autopilot, and act in the same old ways, before they even know what happened, leading to the same old situation. For example, you would probably find it easier to think of your emotions when you get angry at a person, than it is to recall which thoughts began the process of growing angry.

Identify a cue image of the current habit, and write it down in detail in your journal before moving on to the next step.

• Your Ideal Reality: Next, you should take some time to picture your ideal reality or outcome from the changes you're about to make. What, exactly, do you wish for your life to look like? In what specific ways do you want to behave and react? The more intense and clear this image is, the more success you will experience with the method. You may want to be able to climb five flights of stairs without much stress on your body, or envision yourself turning down a second helping of apple pie during the holidays.

You might envision accepting an invitation to your friend's pool party, instead of saying no because you're embarrassed about being seen in a bathing suit. Perhaps you will imagine being able to try on clothes that fit you 10 years ago, and wear them with confidence out in public. Whatever your goal is, make sure you get specific.

Be faithful with your practice of this technique, and remember that the stronger the feelings, and the clearer the image, the better the results will be. You should notice mental and physical changes not long after beginning this new practice.

Technique 3: NLP Visualization to Make Unhealthy Food Unappealing

This next section will guide you through detailed visualization and a step by step process for making junk food unappealing. Does this sound impossible? You might wonder if you can enjoy success with visualization, but this is a technique employed by celebrities, athletes, and average people to learn how to improve in their careers, relax and experience less stress, and accomplish goals. This technique works for quitting smoking, having fewer headaches, and it can work for weight loss too. Using this technique, you will have:

• The Ability to Discern True Hunger: Visualization can help you with telling when you are truly hungry and in need of food, instead of just craving. You may even find that you feel hungry less often and only feel the urge to eat what you actually need. Eating only when you are actually hungry means choosing healthier options, instead of the first junk you come upon.

• More Energy: You can use visualization to feel less lethargic and tired throughout your day. The fact that you will crave junk food less contributes to the rise in energy levels that result from this method.

• Lasting Change: This method does not require forcing yourself into a fitness routine or starving yourself. In fact, once you align your eating habits with the needs of your body, the pounds will come off on their own. Unlike fad diets, this method allows lasting change for your body and lifestyle. Visualization allows your body and mind to work with each other, not against each other.

Steps for Visualizing your Way to a Healthy Weight:

• Envision your Ideal Self: Use visualization to target your issues with weight gain by picturing yourself at your ideal weight and shape. Do you wish to be fit and thin, with visible abs? Then this is what you should picture. Although this may seem crazy or impossible at this stage, don't get hung up on how realistic or unrealistic it is. Concern yourself only with creating a clear picture of the direction you wish to head in. By the law of attraction, focusing on what you want instead of what you don't want will help lead you to become what you are envisioning.

Picturing vivid and clear imagines is the best way to send messages to your subconscious. Studies have shown that when our minds enter into a stage of extreme relaxation, which body-mind practices and visualization bring on, it's in the perfect state for new suggestions. The first step is getting into a calm and relaxed physical and mental state, breathing deeply and slowly, for about 10 minutes. Once you are in this state, picture your image, and make it as vivid as you possibly can.

• Use Images to Lower your Stress Levels: One fact becomes clear when one takes a look at studies on obesity, and this is stress leading to increased weight. When you live a pressured life, your body begins habitually releasing hormones that make your metabolism slower, make you hungry, and lead your body to store fat. You can use visualization to reduce the stress you feel in your life, staying calm through the most hectic parts of your day. Similar to the step detailed above, breathe deeply for about 10 minutes, and once you are in a relaxed state, picture yourself encountering the stresses of your daily life, but staying calm, instead of becoming stressed out.

• Create Alternative Protection for Emotional Issues: Many people store weight on their bodies as a way to protect themselves against emotional difficulty in life. For example, you might have an abusive boss who yells at you a lot, and subconsciously add on weight to create a barrier against this. You may have recently gone through a breakup and turn to food as a comfort and use the weight that stacks on as a way to hide from the pain. What you should do, instead, is figure out what you are using your weight to hide from.

Next, use a visualization of protection to insulate yourself against this old defense mechanism. Breathe slowly and deeply for at least 10 minutes, and once in your relaxed state of mind, picture begin surrounded by a circle or bright light that protects you from your surroundings. Although this is purely mental, you are communicating a message with your subconscious that you are safe and untouchable. Eventually, your mind will fully accept this message and stop using extra weight as a subconscious defense mechanism.

Using the methods listed above, you can start putting your mind's natural power to use, using visualization exercises to get to the root of the issue that has been causing you to gain weight and keep it on. Your body's natural state is fit, thin, and healthy, and it's just a matter of training the rest of you to believe this. Once you mind and subconscious are convinced, your body and habits will follow suit, creating lasting and real change.

Chapter 8: Satisfaction, Not Deprivation

Before we can go further, we have to be able to understand what *satisfaction* and *deprivation* mean.

First of all, satisfaction is the feeling of contentment one gets when they have done or acquired what they wanted. People mostly feel satisfied once they have fed their emotional hunger, even though that satisfaction doesn't last. A person is said to be satisfied when their emotions are over washed by a feeling of fulfillment or contentment

Deprivation, on the other hand, means withholding something from one's self even when it is absolutely necessary. Some say it's an act of self-punishment, especially in the throes of shame and guilt. A person might starve themselves just because they indulged a little too much when they knew they shouldn't have.

Whenever you do something for yourself, something you feel is right for you, something that makes you happy and gives you joy, there is always an accompanying feeling of self-satisfaction. Basically, your mind is telling you that it is pleased with you.

Deprivation mostly accompanies the feeling of satisfaction in emotional eaters. Many of them feel ashamed that they are enjoying anything at all when they do not look good enough, or fit enough. Some seek to deprive themselves after straying from their diet, as if to make up for the little blunder.

It doesn't have to always be that way. You have to feel good about yourself. It's your right, and no one can take it away from you.

Satisfaction is our brain's emotional reward system. That feeling is always there to let you know when you are doing the right things. I should probably point out that feeling satisfied doesn't necessarily mean you have done the right thing. Eating that plate of pasta must have left you feeling satisfied, even when it sabotaged your dietary plans.

Satisfaction is an emotion that is very easy to identify.

When you are going on a diet plan, always aim to arrange it in such a way it doesn't feel like a chore or a trip to the doctor's office. Aim to please yourself, because at the end of the day, it's only your opinion that matters.

Depriving yourself of certain things is also not a solution. In some cases, it can be bad for our health. For example, depriving yourself of food because you over indulged is really not a good idea. Your body needs nutrients to function. What you should do instead is give it more of the right stuff, and less of the bad stuff.

If you care so much about other people's opinions, hear me now: your actions don't affect them. They affect *you*. So, be careful when you feel you need to deprive yourself to fit some ridiculous standard you perceive everyone around you has set for you. Deprivation only ever makes things worse! Not better. I mean, why would you deprive yourself of food when your body needs those nutrients to survive? Without the food, you'd die!

I'm not talking about fasting here. That's different, and deliberate, and borne out of a sheer desire to reset the system. If that's what you're doing then great! Just be sure to follow medical advice while you're at it. But if this is a guilt thing, then you're depriving yourself, and I promise it's a circle that never ends. You're only going to binge again. Your brief moment of satisfaction shouldn't end in endless hours of agony just because you made a mistake. Move on!

Don't Beat Yourself Up

I know there have been a lot of instances where you browbeat yourself before or after you eat something. At that moment, your thoughts are everywhere, and you start to wonder if you really should have eaten what you ate. You wonder what would happen if you eat a certain food. You wonder how to make up for enjoying that juicy burger a little too much. *Need I continue?*

That voice inside your head that brow beats you at every given opportunity is an enemy. An enemy you need to vanquish. This enemy is rooted so deep in your mind it never even occurs to you to question it. You decide to order in a box of pizza after a long day at work and that voice in your head starts to scream and rant after you've had the pizza already. "Pizzas are terrible! They will make you fat! You will never lose weight at this rate! You should have eaten a bowl of fruit salad instead! Now we're going to have to fix this! What do we do? No food for the next five months!"

Do Away with Labels

Yes, we know certain foods really are good or bad for you. But! We need to help you actually be able to do away with guilt. See, once you stop feeling guilty for eating something, you're better able to make better decisions and choices for your body. So how do we achieve this?

Don't label your food. I t may seem counterintuitive, but don't. At best, just tell yourself, "I eat this, I don't eat that." Don't be forceful about it. Just gently tell yourself that when dealing with temptations. .

You see, putting good or bad labels on foods stops you from actually enjoying what you are eating, whether or not it really is good or bad! Once you have already decided a food is bad, you will be engulfed by a feeling of guilt and shame which in most cases leads you to deprive yourself of something else you like as punishment. You'll become so obsessed with what to eat or not eat that all that analysis paralysis will just leave your brain fried. Remember what you do when you're overwhelmed? You go for the easiest option. And that just keeps you stuck in emotional eating mode.

Emotional eating usually makes this even worse and feelings of guilt or shame easily result in self-derision, self-loathing, self-deceiving, ruin, hopelessness, and shame. To rid yourself of that feeling of having lost all control of yourself, you start to feel like you have to make up for it using self-destructive behaviors and self-imposed rules. You start to feel bad and worthless if you wolf down a snack just before dinner. You feel bad for eating when you feel like you should be exercising. After all, that's what others are doing

You are not them!

These feelings of guilt and self-deprivation are always as a result of fear of failure. This fear may push you to punish yourself with destructive behaviors like drug abuse, smoking, alcohol abuse, compulsive exercising and so on.

Never Enough

What people do not know is that these feelings aren't necessarily related to food. They are just as a result of one's inability to accept and love yourself unconditionally, because that nagging and annoying voice in your head keeps telling you that you are not good enough, pretty enough, smart enough or funny enough.

These feelings of guilt or shame after eating something "bad" or doing something you feel you shouldn't have is just your way of dealing with the feeling. If you start to feel bad about everything that enters your mouth, before long, what you eat will be what defines your mood.

Man, Know Thyself

Observing your behavioral pattern is an important part of your recovery. The rules, the "good" and "bad" labels, the deprivation and self-destructive derision stop you from seeking any form of help. This is because you have become your own judge and jury system. Sorting out the jungle that Is your feelings, learning how to enjoy food again is one of the surest ways to recovery.

More often than not, we eat based on our feelings, and a lot of times, food affects the way we feel. Eating goes way beyond physical hunger, even though, granted, we eat when we are hungry. We eat to fill out bellies. We eat to be satisfied; to have feelings of pleasure and fulfillment. We have to understand the reasoning behind our food choices to be able to feel satisfied with our choice.

How to Be Satisfied with Your Food

With such a wide range of foods to choose from, how does one get satisfaction from food? Most importantly, feelings of satisfaction differ from person to person. While a person might derive pleasure and satisfaction from eating a home-cooked meal in a cost environment, another might enjoy eating a bit of chocolate while working.

Consuming food is a repetitive action. It's one our survival depends on. A person may crave something sugary, but still won't get that satisfaction from eating a very succulent apple. One might want to go for something even more sugary than that. So, a piece of chocolate would seem a better option to that person, as opposed to the apple, just to fill that void or hole they may feel in their emotions.   Although a person might feel some satisfaction from doing this, feelings of shame or guilt follow closely behind.

Eating to cope can increase negative responses and emotions towards food, especially in the end. The cause of the stress is temporarily forgotten because we are more focused on our fat, oil, and sugar-filled food choices.   Regular consumption of unhealthful foods can result in unnecessary weight gain, poor self-esteem, and bad body image. When we have negative feelings about ourselves, it speeds up the process of guilt and shame, and accelerates the movement of the cycle.

Attaining Maximum Satisfaction

If we are trying to get the ultimate satisfaction, we have to eradicate every feeling of guilt, shame, self-derision, deprivation, and self-loathing following each meal. Although food should not be used as a reward system all the time, a glass of wine during Thanksgiving or eating a slice of cake on your birthday is perfectly acceptable.

So, no need to be mad at yourself!

If you know you will always be racked with guilt whenever you eat something, try to find something you can eat without being filled with shame. Some people can eat nuts without being filled with guilt. They are perfectly healthy. Having a healthy relationship with the foods you eat is very important as it keeps us in touch with our external and internal environment. It helps us deal with our muddled emotions and find a way to reduce disordered patterns and thoughts.

The purpose of that small voice in our head is to whisper needed suggestions that can help us make better choices, but it can be a bit warped, twisted into a little monster of criticism from our guilt. We have to always bear it at the back of our minds eating that bit of chocolate fudge at the end of a stressful day will not make the day any less stressful than it actually was. It won't even give your body the essential nutrients that it needs. *So why bother?*

You have to be able to understand your body's language, and be cognizant of any signal your body gives, especially it's yelling at you, "Hey, buddy, I am full!" Understanding these signals help us make better choices towards better health and general wellness, as opposed to guilt and deprivation.

Chapter 9: The Repercussions of Emotional Eating

We have already ascertained emotional eating can have very dangerous consequences to our physical health, mental health, even our social life.

One study was carried out which proved that there is no such thing as a "comfort food."

What?

With your level of intelligence and intellectual ability, you must have already noticed that the so called "comfort foods" we have around provides little comfort.

Comfort Foods Are Not Real

An experiment was carried out on a group of self-acclaimed chocolate lovers. The researchers induced stress in the participants by having them all insert their hands in cold water for some time. It's probably not you would call stress... after all, it is not as back-breaking as the stress you get from work challenges and all, but the body reacts the same way to all types of stress.

Anyway, the participants were then given hand grips so the researchers could measure how much effort they put into gripping them in order to get a piece of chocolate. It may sound a little bit silly to you, but the results were anything but.

Stress As A Motivator

The truth is stress makes us crave rewards and pushes us to get them. How many times have you found yourself motivating yourself to finish that last bout of vigorous exercise so you could get yourself a good cold glass of water? Or have you ever promised yourself a big piece of chocolate if you were able to finish a task you set for yourself? Then you can relate to what I'm saying.

This research also shows we do not always derive the amount of pleasure from the reward as we expect. This study was conducted at the University of Geneva, Switzerland. So you know they must have used only the best quality chocolate.

No matter how tempting it may seem, emotional eating doesn't really deal with stress the way we'd like it to. It just postpones it for another time. SO rather than grab a bar of chocolate, lace up your shoes and go for a jog! Work up a proper sweat!

Working out is a great way to relieve yourself of stress. By the time you're all done, nice and sweaty, you're going to find you've completely forgotten you had a craving to begin with.

Effects of Emotional Eating

Emotional eating has become one of a very long list of problems which not only mess up our psyche, but wreaks havoc on our physical health, too. People have been known to eat for many different reasons besides hunger.

Emotional eating can stem from many issues. Some people have even claimed to develop the habit as a side effect of some medicines such as birth control.

There are a lot of side effects to emotional eating, both physical and emotional. We shall see a few of them before we look into healthier methods of feeding. I know you already know a few of these detrimental repercussions of giving in to emotional hunger, but let's just go over some of the major ones really quick.

• _Feeling shame or guilt._ After whatever emotional crisis we are going through, we are usually flooded by a huge wave of shame or guilt, especially when we realise how much we have chowed in our bid to deal with this emotional crisis. This feeling of shame also has the ability to further plunge us in a gaping emotional hole, causing us to eat again, and again, and again, and that vicious cycle continues.

• *Bouts of nausea.* A lot of people who suffer from panic attacks or anxiety attacks are usually comforted by the "feelings" they have in their stomach which they mistaken as need for food. This often results in bouts of nausea after they have over indulged. These bouts of nausea are sometimes quite severe, and sometimes these symptoms may persist even after days of having indulged. This usually puts them off other foods for some time until the process is repeated again.

• *Health complications.* There are a lot of health problems related to repetitive indulgence in emotional eating. Health conditions like type 2 diabetes, elevated blood pressure, extreme fatigue. and obesity are all examples of how our bodies bear the brunt of our overindulgence.

• *Lack of focus.* People often see food as a method of distracting them from their problems. A most effective way of dealing with emotional eating is finding another distraction. Some people start to feel lost, or they lose focus when they do not have food to soothe them. It is a bad habit, and if left unchecked, it can leave a person regularly distracted. If you always find yourself reaching for food to distract yourself, then find something else to distract you. Try distractions that have definite health benefits such as bicycling or going for a walk in the park, or even going out with a couple of friends. While it may seem the main problem is you have no control over what you eat, emotional eating actually starts with our lack of control over our emotions.

- *Excessive weight gain.* This is one of the first noticeable side effects of emotional eating. Excessive weight puts a lot of pressure on our bones and muscles. You start to feel muscle and joint pain. You also feel tired, irritated, and in extreme cases, you may not be to bear your body's weight.

- Lack of confidence and self-esteem

People have undergone excessive weight gain tend to worry a lot about physical appearances and social acceptance. This causes a steady decline in their self-esteem and confidence. They tend to deprive themselves of the food they feel make them fat and in turn tend to eat more from hunger

- Emotional distress

When a person ends up realising the consequences of their over indulgence, it's usually too late. This further depresses them and causes undue distress. You start to have feelings of paranoia and start to see snide looks where there are none. In the long run, you still continue to overeat as a way to soothe your distress. When you eventually get depressed, you eat more and more to counter the effect of these negative emotions

- Increased metabolic imbalance

After some time, you start to have metabolic imbalances due to fluctuations in electrolyte levels which result in increased levels of anxiety, loneliness, and frustration. At this point you find it difficult to perform simple tasks. The sight of food makes you more and more insecure about yourself.

- Affects your relationships. Emotional eating affects our relationship with family, relatives, and friends. This is usually because food and the need for the next "fix" becomes your major concern, so you have no time for any other thing. After all, that burger has to come out of your mouth before you can talk to anybody!

• Digestive problems. Once your diet starts to consist only of high fat junk food and high calorie foods, you open yourself to different kinds of gastrointestinal problems which can cause serious damage to your digestive system. You become very prone to different kinds of allergic reactions because your body can no longer deal with the large quantities of junk you now consume very regularly. Your system might not be able to cope if you persist with such a really bad diet.

• High cholesterol levels. Emotional eating makes you very susceptible to diseases that are caused by high cholesterol and high blood sugar levels due to excessive consumption of food.

• Organ Malfunction. Another health risk of emotional eating excesses is organ malfunction. Your liver, kidney, stomach, and other organs in the body which handle digestion and nutrient assimilation then become extremely prone to diseases and disorders.

• Skin related problems. When we consume too much high fat junk foods, we increase the oil levels in our body, which can lead to many skin-related problems like acne and pimples.

• Acid reflux. Excessive emotional eating can increase acidity levels in our bodies which causes a serious digestive condition called acid reflux.

• Poor oral hygiene. People who overeat focus so much on putting food in their mouth that they rarely have the time to brush and clean their teeth properly. I don't have to tell you the sort of havoc that wreaks on their dental health. And since oral hygiene has been linked to a lot of serious diseases, then that just makes things worse for the emotional overeater.

• Drowsiness. Emotional eaters are mostly so caught up in food that sometimes they lose their train of thought and focus. Most times they are found dozing off at the place where they just, sometimes with their hands still in the pack of chips.

If you want to avoid all of this, then you had better implement the plans and tips I've given you in this book so far! No time like the present to get started.

Chapter 10: Take Action, Take Back Your Life

So you've identified your emotions and are now working on understanding and potentially coming to peace with them. Now it's time for action, which admittedly can be just as hard as coming to terms with why you binge. This is because taking action to stop binge eating comes down to a simple choice: do you or do you not want to stop binge eating? You've picked up this book, so there is definitely some desire to stop. Now make a decision and keep on moving forward. Remember, you can do this.

Jump Start Your Morning

The important thing to remember when trying to form any new habit is that you have to wake up with the right mindset. Putting it off and saying you'll take care of that after breakfast, or lunch, or next weekend will only help to enable the behavior you are trying to get rid of. So when you wake up, it is good to not only have a specific mindset, but to have a plan.

Instead of waking up and grabbing whatever food is in the cupboards for breakfast, plan your meal the day prior. Figure out what you would like for the entire day: meals, snacks, and dessert. Then when you go out the door in the morning, you'll have had a healthy breakfast and be bringing the food you'll need throughout the day to work with you. This way, you'll avoid the random snack at coffee shops on the way to work and the vending machines once you get there.

If your binge eating runs in the cycle of binging, self-shaming, and then punishing yourself through a lack of food, it may be a good idea to throw out your weight scale. Not having a constant reminder that you are not at whatever weight you want to be (and seriously consider if that is a healthy weight and how you are approaching reaching it), will help you to start the morning thinking about how you feel physically and mentally, rather than how you look. Pay attention to whether you feel well rested and if movement feels like a chore, as well as how you regard yourself in the morning. Have compassion for yourself physically, emotionally, and mentally right from the start; this will make it easier to continue caring for yourself throughout the day.

Another way to help yourself is to slow down when eating. Many who suffer from BED report that they eat uncommonly fast, which aids both the extreme consumption of food and helps to distract the individual from the problem at hand. So next time you sit down to a meal, particularly if you are by yourself, try setting down your utensils after every bite. Force yourself to slow down, breathe, and digest your food. This may also help you to notice when you are full and stop eating before the feeling becomes uncomfortable.

It is also imperative to remember to forgive yourself. Sometimes you'll have a bad day. That doesn't mean you should plan for one; certainly "cheat" days will do you no favors, but nobody is perfect, so don't expect yourself to be. If you slip and find yourself halfway through a bag of chips, then throw them out, forgive yourself, and start over. Eventually, through a lot of hard work, it will get easier.

Eating Healthier

This is often a dreaded topic. Many people detest the thought of switching out their white rice for brown, but this issue of eating in a much more nutrient-conscious way actually starts at a more basic level.

The first thing to do is begin every week with a specific meal plan in mind. Try buying some cookbooks or going online to find inspirational recipes that don't seem foreign but are still a departure from less healthy eating habits (magazines like *Bon Appetite* and *Cooking Light* have wonderful recipes that are both delicious and healthy). Jot down a few of these, attempting to choose a collection of recipes with the same core ingredients so as to avoid excess food that will go bad (like fresh herbs) or become target for a session of binge eating.

After you have selected your recipes, create a detailed grocery list. Be sure to specify what every item should be, so there is no room for questionable items, i.e. "snack." If you don't do this, there is a higher chance that you'll grab a couple of items because you either don't know what you want or you want everything. By replacing "snack" with "blueberries" you may avoid grabbing three different chip assortments. However, if you get home and realize you have not held true to the list, then simply throw the binging item out. And of course, always follow the cardinal grocery-shopping rule: never shop when you are hungry.

Once you have done your shopping, set about prepping all of the food for the week. This should be done immediately after shopping and you should give yourself a day to do it, usually a weekend. It may also be wise to have someone present while you conduct the shopping and cooking. Having a witness could be helpful in preventing a binging episode and may allow you to place all of your concentration on the task at hand instead of providing opportunity to binge eat. Try to make this ritual a fun event that you look forward to every week.

Following completing the week's cooking, separate all of your meals into separate containers, label them, and then refrain from buying any more food for the rest of the week. If you hold true to this, it will help to space out food portions appropriately, taking into account the amount of nutrients your body requires each day. Later on in the week, if you feel the desire to binge, remind yourself that the only food in the house has been allotted to specific meals and that you cannot spend any more money on food for the week.

Keep in mind that eating in a health-conscious way is not about losing weight, although it will certainly help you to do so. Rather, consuming healthy food is a crucial key to having a long and productive life. Substituting refined sugars for natural sweeteners like Stevia can help to reduce the risk of cancer and diabetes. Upping the amount of fish you eat every week and reducing red meat intake will fuel your body with healthy fats and oils without negatively contributing to cholesterol. If you are not sure how to change your eating habits, research diets such as the Mediterranean diet, which emphasizes healthy food substitutions and large, daily quantities of fruits and vegetables.

While changing your diet is a necessary recovery factor, don't be intimidated by the word diet. Modifications in eating habits are not about punishment and the exclusion of foods, but the improvement of health through change. To motivate yourself to eat healthier foods, focus on trying new things and how the healthier foods will make you feel. Lastly, speak to a therapist about the changes you are making and how it may alter your relationships with food and yourself.

Exercise

For many bingers, exercise must begin at a very basic level. Since food binging frequently leads to obesity, it is important to treat the body gently. You may have the motivation to run ten miles but your body will collapse because it is not used to or cannot handle being put under that kind of stress. So instead, start with very little things. Instead of taking the escalator, walk up the stairs. Additionally, if you are someone who greatly enjoys television, cut down to a show or two and use your free time to take a walk and stretch instead.

Another way to start off the morning right in regards to exercise is to buy a small pair of dumbbells (2-5 pounds.) and place them directly in front of your bed, even to the point of placing them next to where your feet land when getting out of bed in the morning. This way, exercise will be one of the first things to enter your mind. Try doing a variety of exercises with them, whether that is sitting in your bed doing a few curls, or more advanced exercises such as holding them while doing squats or placing them on your stomach during crunches. Remember, everyone starts off at a different point and so it is important not to compare yourself to others. Despite how it feels, your muscles, aided by a nutritional diet and plenty of water, will begin to strengthen and eventually you will be able to move on to more advanced levels.

Exercise also works wonderfully as a way to keep your mind off of eating. Again, it is not wise to trade one addiction for another (and extraneous exercise can certainly fall under that category), but exercise can serve as another distraction. Instead of reaching for a box of donuts, go for a walk instead.

While exercising can seem like an ordeal, it is important to remember that it does not have to be a chore. Many simple stretching exercises can be done while watching television, lying on the floor, sitting, or standing. Visit the link from Fit City Aitkin in the footnote for tips.[6]

Here is an incredibly helpful last tip: don't exercise alone. If you are someone who is used to a moderate amount of physical activity but absolutely loathes going to the gym, consider signing up for a class with a friend. There are a million activities out there, from dance to self-defense, which can serve as the exercise your body needs. And while it can be difficult sometimes to work on fitness with a friend, especially if the friend is already immersed in physical health, you would be amazed at the power of obligation. Set up a time, say three days a week, in which you are scheduled to meet a friend and exercise, whether that is at the park, gym, or home. You'll find it is much more difficult to avoid working out when you've already promised your time to someone than if you are home alone and there is a good book on the table. Additionally, the encouragement you receive from being with a friend can be helpful. Those positive emotions created by encouragement and knowing that you are doing something about your predicament may help to combat the feelings that lead you to binge.

Step-by-Step

Making a lifestyle change can be daunting, and for good reason; it takes a tremendous amount of focus and self-analyzing. It is far too easy to become dissuaded from the true goal of recovering from BED, which is to be healthy emotionally, mentally, and physically, and instead focus only on changing one's exterior. This severe misstep can make recovery even more difficult, and is a mistake easily made when attempting a lifestyle change. This is due to the huge scope of recovery. When faced with the obstacles of overcoming BED, it isn't difficult to become overwhelmed and fall into a state of hopelessness. So instead of driving blind, come up with a step-by-step plan to help you on your way to recovery and to build a foundation of support for once you get there.

Think of it this way: if you take a road trip to a foreign city across state lines, you need to have a game plan. Know how far you need to go each day and where your checkpoints are. Figure out what to do if the car breaks down a.k.a. you have a relapse, and who to seek help from. Once you get to the foreign city, figure out how to survive there. In other words, have a game plan for your recovery, stick to it the best that you can, and learn how to keep healthy once you've achieved your health. Most importantly though, remember that this game plan is merely an outline for your recovery. Tailor it to your specific needs and make any and all necessary changes while your plan is in motion.

Chapter 11: Respect Your Hunger

Keep your body sustained organically with sufficient vitality and starches.

Else, you can trigger a base drive to gorge. When you arrive right now of unnecessary craving, all expectations of moderate, cognizant eating are short lived and superfluous.

Figuring out how to respect this first organic sign sets the stage for revamping trust with yourself and nourishment.

Mechanisms That Trigger Eating

Regardless of whether you are a constant dieter, ground-breaking natural systems are activated when your body doesn't get the vitality from nourishment that it needs. It's no mishap that nourishment is incorporated as one of the major human needs in Maslow's Hierarchy of Needs—a model that positions human needs, recommending that specific fundamental needs should be met before you can proceed to satisfy increasingly complex ones. Nourishment and vitality are so fundamental to the endurance of the human species that on the off chance that we don't eat enough we set off an organic wire that turns on our eating drive both physically and mentally.

The craving drive is really a mind-body association. Eating is critical to the point that the nerve cells of hunger are situated in the nerve center area of the mind.

An assortment of organic sign triggers eating. What numerous people accept to be an issue of self-discipline is rather an organic drive. The power and force of the natural eating drive ought not to be thought little of.

The neurochemicals from the cerebrum arrange our eating conduct with our body's organic need. Through a perplexing arrangement of substance and neural input, the cerebrum screens the vitality needs of all our body frameworks, minute to minute.

What's more, it makes exceptionally unequivocal compound mandates as what exactly we ought to eat. Fasting or limiting is especially unfavorable to craving control. It basically turns on the neurochemical switches that incite us to eat.

Numerous examinations have demonstrated that bringing down body weight by nourishment limitation furthermore, dieting has neither rhyme nor reason metabolically or to our mind science.

Actually, it's counterproductive. The organic synthetics that direct hunger likewise legitimately influence temperaments and perspective, our physical vitality and our sexual experiences.

Most analysts concur that there are both complex natural and mental instruments that impact our eating.

Honor your hunger

The initial step to recovering the universe of typical eating, free of dieting what's more, nourishment stress, is to respect your natural appetite. Your body needs to know reliably that it will approach nourishment—that dieting and hardship have stopped, unequivocally. Something else, your science will continuously be accessible as needs be, prepared to deflect a willful nourishment hardship.

Your body should be naturally reconditioned. Diet after diet has shown your body that individual starvations are visit, so it should remain on protect.

Keep in mind, starvations and nourishment deficiencies have consistently existed, indeed, even in our cutting edge times. Our bodies are still organically prepared to endure starvations through bringing down our vitality prerequisites, expanding natural synthetic compounds that trigger our eating drive, etc.

It is a lot simpler to quit eating when your body isn't starving. For model, envision you are in a room and offer a destitute youngster a plate of treats. You tell the youngster that she can have just a single treat. You exit the room and disregard the kid with the entire plate. What might the hungry kid do? Eat every one of the treats (and lick the pieces), obviously.

In any case, if the youngster realized that treats (or some other nourishment) were constantly accessible whenever hungry, the extraordinary drive to eat would be enormously decreased.

The equivalent is valid for dieters.

For instance, Barbara generally kept herself in a ravenous state. She as it were enabled herself to eat when very eager. By her own definition, on the off chance that she enabled herself to eat when essentially eager, yet not avaricious, she thought she was overeating. However in light of the fact that her meaning of "typical" yearning was being insatiable, her eating would waver from gala to starvation cycles.

Yearning SILENCE

Imagine a scenario in which you don't feel hunger any longer, or don't generally have a clue what the delicate vibe of yearning feels like? Would you be able to get it back? Truly. On the whole we should take a gander at a few reasons why yearning might be hushed.

• Numbing. A number of people have learned throughout the years to suppress, or deflect cravings for food by going to without calorie drinks, for example, diet soft drinks, espresso, and tea. The fluid in the stomach incidentally deceives the gastric component into a feeling of totality.

• Dieting. Dieters get so used to denying their appetite that it moves toward becoming simple to block it out. In the end, when craving comes thumping on their internal entryway and there is no reaction, the thumping, or rather the stomach thundering, stops.

• Chaos. It's anything but difficult to stifle hunger or overlook it, when you are caught up with putting out the flames throughout your life or employment. In the event that this is a ceaseless example, craving may gradually blur.

• Skipping Breakfast. A portion of our customers skip breakfast in the first part of the day, since they state it keeps them feeling hungrier the remainder of the day or on the other hand since they're in a rush. However yearning is a typical, invited body signal that ought to be grasped. It's an indication that you are getting back in contact with your body's needs. But since these customers fear their appetite, they react by not eating breakfast the following morning— which rehashes the endless loop of craving quietness.

Chapter 12: Make Peace with Food

Call a détente; stop the nourishment battle! Give yourself unrestricted authorization to eat. On the off chance that you disclose to yourself that you can't or shouldn't have a specific nourishment, it can prompt serious sentiments of hardship that incorporate with wild longings and, frequently, gorging.

When you at last "surrender" to your prohibited nourishments, eating will be knowledgeable about such power, it typically brings about Last Supper overeating and overpowering blame.

The Peace Process

Making harmony with nourishment means permitting all food sources into your eating world, with the goal that a decision for chocolate turns out to be genuinely equivalent to the decision for a peach. While for quite a long time numerous wellbeing experts have concurred that there ought to be no taboo nourishments, not many will take care of business furthermore, state, eat anything you desire. In the end there is a farthest point forced. Furthermore, knowing there is a point of confinement can at present give a nourishment desire of sorts—better eat it now!

Unexpectedly, when you really realize you can eat anything you desire, the exceptional inclination to eat significantly lessens.

The best method to impart faith in this reality is to experience eating the very nourishments you preclude! It winds up plainly obvious that you can "handle" these nourishments, or even better, that they have no enchantment hang on you or your self-discipline.

Amusingly, numerous, of our customers find that the very nourishments they denied and ached for, / are never again attractive once they can be eaten openly. Again and again, we hear accounts of how when they were genuinely permitted to eat certain nourishments, they found, incredibly, that they truly didn't care for them to start with!

Fears That Hold You Back

Indeed, even customers who come prepared to quit any pretense of dieting have a solid opposition against eating whatever they truly need. They are alarmed. While they feel good figuring out how to respect their craving, they are prepared to jolt out the entryway when we talk about giving unqualified authorization to eat what they like.

"If people are so hesitant to progress to this piece of the Intuitive Eating process, for what reason do we demand that it must be investigated? Sanctioning nourishment is the basic advance in changing your association with nourishment. It liberates you to react to internal eating signals that have been covered by negative contemplations and blame emotions about eating.

 In the event that you don't genuinely accept that you can eat whatever nourishment you like, you will keep on inclination denied, at last indulge, and be obstructed from inclination happy with your eating.

What's more, when you are not fulfilled, you will be lurking in the shadows for additional food when you realize the nourishment will be there and permitted, for quite a while, it doesn't turn out to be so imperative to have it. Nourishment loses its capacity.

Five Steps to Making Peace with Food

Remember as you read through these means that it's alright to continue at a pace with which you are agreeable. There is no compelling reason to feel overpowered by setting off to the supermarket and purchasing each and every prohibited nourishment—we find that is too huge a stage and a bit much.

It requires some investment to develop trust in yourself. Before you continue, if it's not too much trouble is certain that you are reliably regarding your craving. An insatiable individual is bound to gorge paying little heed to their aim.

1. Focus on nourishments that intrigue to you and make a rundown of them.

2. Put a check by the nourishments you really eat, at that point circle remaining nourishments that you've been limiting.

3. Give yourself consent to eat one prohibited nourishment from your rundown, at that point go to the market and purchase this nourishment, or request it at an eatery.

4. Check in with yourself to check whether the nourishment tastes on a par with you envisioned. In the event that you find that you truly like it, keep on giving yourself consent to purchase or request it.

5. Ensure that you keep enough of the nourishment in your kitchen so that you realize it will be there in the event that you need it. Or on the other hand if that appears to be excessively startling, go to an eatery and

request the specific nourishment as regularly as you like.

When you've made harmony with one nourishment, proceed with your rundown until every one of the nourishments are attempted, assessed, and liberated. In the event that your rundown is very enormous, which is conceivable, we have discovered that you don't need to involvement every single nourishment recorded. Or maybe, what is significant is that you proceed with this procedure until you really realize you can eat what you need.

You will arrive at a point where you don't need to encounter the "verification" by eating.

In the event that these means appear a lot to deal with this moment, don't stress.

Perhaps you can call a truce, which is alright—it's encouraging. The following section will give you a few instruments to enable you to release up with your nourishment.

Similarly the same number of harmony bargains require a group of moderators—and time— the following section will assist you find amazing partners with helping keep the harmony with nourishment.

Chapter 13: Learning to Move Your Body

In this chapter, we move on to discussing a different aspect of your relationship with your body—specifically body movement. I use "body movement" instead of "exercise" because I know that the "e word" has lots of negative connotations. It has been co-opted by the diet industry just as food has—in other words, used only in the service of trying to get you to lose weight. No wonder just thinking about exercise may send you into a fit of resistance or may make you feel guilty that you're not doing enough or not doing the right kind—at least according to all the experts.

Just as I encouraged you to question the conventional wisdom that says you have to be thin to be healthy, or that some foods are "bad foods" and you should only eat "good foods," I am encouraging you now to turn your inner skeptic loose on the field of exercise and all its attendant "expert" advice. To begin, I will discuss the problems with exercise prescriptions that often keep heavier people standing on the sidelines. Then you will learn how to remove your personal exercise blocks and find enjoyment in moving your body again. This chapter will help you embrace your intuitive connection with your body's natural need to be in motion. This chapter is about allowing you to stretch and move your way beyond the yoke of exercise as a mandate for weight loss and into a new relationship with movement as the body's birthright.

To start our skeptic's journey to body movement, I'd like you to take a little trip down memory lane in the exercise below.

Exercise: How I Learned to Crawl and Walk

You may want to pull out an old photo album and choose three or more pictures of yourself at different ages, from toddler to age five, for example. Start by sitting in a comfortable chair with your feet flat on the floor. Take three deep breaths, breathing in through your nose and out through your mouth. Now bring your attention to the sensation of your breath moving through your entire body, from the top of your scalp to the soles of your feet. Imagine that your breath is moving through your body in the same way your body moves through life. You can imagine your breath dancing, swirling, stomping, and gliding through all the cells and organs in your body and as part of what connects your body to the vital energy that is life itself. Bring your attention now to the sensations in your feet. Now start to remember yourself as a child, thinking of the pictures you've found. If you have any issues with remembering yourself as a child, you can think of another child to use as a surrogate for this exercise. This may be your own child, a niece or nephew, or the child of a friend. As you go through the exercise, keep breathing and keep your attention on your feet.

Looking at each picture or thinking of a mental picture of yourself or of another beloved child, write down any memories you have of moving your body when you were a kid. Maybe one of your pictures shows you in motion, or you may have a mental image of yourself in movement. Maybe there's a family story you recall about your being active or liking certain activities when you were younger. If you are using a surrogate child, think of all the ways in which this child moves his or her body. The idea here is to capture the essence of how children (and you specifically) are in movement. Paint a picture that comes to life for you. (Example: When I was a little boy, I used to wear capes and pretend I was a superhero. My mother has lots of pictures of me with towel capes, jumping off of benches and pretending to fly or running in the wind with the cape billowing out behind me. Later, there are lots of pictures of me climbing things. I didn't like traditional sports, but I loved doing cartwheels on the front lawn, swinging in the tire swing in our yard, and playing hide-and-seek in the bamboo forest in my backyard.)

See if you can imagine the feeling of being in movement when you were a child, and describe that feeling. (Example: I felt so free when I was running through the grass in my bare feet or when I would go swimming with my father and he would throw me off his shoulders into the pool. I remember laughing so hard I was hiccoughing when I would ride my bike down a hill, going as fast as I could on a dare from my brother. I felt excited and carefree!)

Now ask yourself what made moving your body feel the way you described above. (Example: I felt free because it felt so natural to be doing what I was doing. No one had to tell me I was doing it right or wrong. I was happy because I was doing what I wanted and loved to do.)

Rediscovering the Natural Joy of Movement

You may be lucky enough to enjoy exercise—even if you are in a bigger body. You may have continued to play a sport you enjoy, or you may have the discipline of a marine drill sergeant and just make yourself do what you think you need to do. To you, I say: "Keep up the good work!" Maybe reading this chapter will help you encourage or be less impatient with friends or family members who don't feel the same way you do about exercise. But if you have food and body image issues, you may struggle with exercise. To you, I say: "Don't throw the baby out with the bath water." What I mean by that is don't let the voices of ex-coaches, parents, peers who teased you, or anyone else who robbed you of the joy of being in motion take away the pleasure inherent in moving your body. Don't let the voices of experts who told you that you will only lose weight by doing certain exercises stay in your head. Kick out of your mind anyone who told you, as Carol was told, that you couldn't do a sport or an activity you wanted to do because of your size! Let's bring the play back into movement and get rid of the idea that exercise is something you have to do. As a child, I remember spending all day every day "exercising" in the community pool in my neighborhood—but really all I was doing was playing with my friends. I remember riding my bike up and down hills trying to catch up with my brothers on their bikes. That could have been considered exercise, but to me it felt like just plain fun. Just as you can learn to eat with joy, you can also reclaim your right to move your body with joy. Moving your body is a natural desire that you have, or at least had when you were younger. For example, babies are in motion all the time, exploring their hands, trying to put their feet in their mouths, and trying to roll over—even when they don't know how. Toddlers start to stand up, eventually let go of coffee tables, and try to walk and then run as soon as they are able. Every time they fall down, they get up and do it again. Why? Because this desire to move the body is hardwired into our genes, and it takes a lot to make moving the body feel like something we have to do rather than something we want to do. In the exercise below, let's examine some of the ways in which your natural desire to move may have been corrupted to make you feel as though you need to "exercise."

Exercise: Exercise Messages

List below messages you got about exercise, body size, or weight. These could have come from family members, coaches, teachers, friends, or magazines and media sources. (Examples: You can't lose weight by swimming. Or My physical education teacher told me I wasn't going to be a good basketball player. He meant I was too fat to be good.)

Describe below all the "exercises" you have tried to lose weight and what the results were, along with how you felt about doing these exercises. (Example: With every diet I go on, I try to do the StairMaster because I know it burns a lot of calories. I literally hate the StairMaster! Sometimes I'd lose weight, but most of the time, I'd get so frustrated with doing it that I would quit.)

Exercise:

How I felt doing this exercise:

How this worked for me:

Exercise:

How I felt doing this exercise:

How this worked for me:

Exercise:

How I felt doing this exercise:

How this worked for me:

Look at your answers to the questions above and see what insights and conclusions you can garner from your history of exercise. (Example: I've never felt like I was very athletic. Because of this, I've always had to force myself to exercise and mainly only do it when I'm trying to lose weight. It's not a pleasant experience for me.)

Good work! You may be thinking that no matter how hard exercising is for you, you still need to do it in order to be healthy and to reach a healthy weight. After all, exercise is good for you just like vegetables are good for you. Right? I would beg to disagree. You don't need to do exercise you hate in order to be healthy. Let's look at this a little more closely.

I Really Don't Need to Exercise?

I want to make the distinction again and again in this chapter between exercise and body movement. Exercise science is used to bury you in scientific information, such as how many calories an activity burns and how many minutes of each activity it takes to lose a certain amount of weight. Just as nutrition science has created a lot of food confusion, exercise science has turned our body's natural desire to be in motion into an experience that feels a lot like boot camp. And by the way, there are actually exercise regimens called boot camp, which promise to whip you into shape whether you like it or not.

When Joyful Body Movement Is Not Good for You

Body movement is not good for you when you don't do it. This is the most important take-home message from this chapter. If you don't move your body, you can't reap all the health benefits available to you no matter what size you are. Remember, it's not about doing something you don't like or forcing yourself to be active doing something you were told you "should" do. This whole chapter is about you rediscovering how natural it is to be in motion. When you read the examples of moderate-intensity exercise above, were you surprised that you could obtain health benefits and live longer by gardening or playing golf? Other examples include actively playing with your children, shoveling light snow, canoeing, and hand-washing a car. There are also jobs that include this type of health-promoting physical activity, such as waiting tables, working on a farm, picking fruits or vegetables, or delivering mail. Vigorous activities that you've been led to believe are the only ones that improve your health and well-being such as jogging, using a StairMaster, biking fast or uphill, and swimming laps are also available to you if you want to do them. But the bottom line is that the only "should" you need pay attention to is the importance of finding an activity you love and want to do, and sticking with it. Some physical activity is much better than none, and if you find a starting point doing something you love, you can build from there. For example, I took up tae kwon do and eventually traveled to Korea to study with my teacher's eighty-year-old teacher, ultimately getting a black belt. Trying something new brought me back to that feeling I had as a child that I was a physical being and that I loved moving my body. I just had to be open to choosing other ways besides the traditional exercises to do that. One of my clients began doing ballroom dancing and now competes all over the country. Another loves swimming laps in her mother's pool for an hour a day in the summer. Another has picked up weight lifting. Yet another client takes three to five yoga classes a week. Another does bike racing in the mountains and extreme bike rides (over fifty miles) with her husband. These are all people who are in bigger bodies who are doing something they love.

Exercise: I Can't Exercise Because...

If you've never been able to effectively initiate or sustain regular physical activity, it may be for some of the reasons listed below. See which you identify with and read the responses to each. Below each reason, write down any insights you have about how these apply to you.

I feel embarrassed by my size and don't want to exercise in public. This is a very valid concern experienced frequently by individuals in larger bodies. But there are always things you can do to make yourself more comfortable with your preferred form of exercise. If you would like to try yoga, for example, but are afraid you'll feel uncomfortable in a class setting, you could take an individual lesson. After one or two private lessons, you may find yourself less embarrassed. Or consider beginning with a simple walking program, building your confidence until you feel ready to join a gym. You can also ask a trusted friend to go with you to the gym or to a dance class so you won't feel so insecure.

But I invite you to go beyond simple solutions to claim your right and privilege—no matter your size—to move your body, just as I advise you to participate more in life. I understand that being bold is not always easy, so you might need to work your way up to it. What I know from experience is that many of my overweight clients are hiding their enthusiasm for life, their creativity, and their natural gifts behind their weight. I encourage you to express yourself by allowing your body to move, dance, do a downward dog pose in yoga, or swim to your heart's content. Every time you step out and express yourself, it will become easier. It will also make it easier for the next heavy person to join your gym or participate in your yoga class.

How does this apply to you? How can you relate? What are you moved to do about this issue so that you can move your body with joy?

I have health problems, and every time I exercise, I have pain, injuries, or other symptoms. This can be a very real problem. If your motivation is strong but you are experiencing pain or other unpleasant symptoms after you exercise, I recommend that you work with a skilled personal trainer or physical therapist to ensure you are exercising safely. If you find that both motivation and physical limitations are at play, you may have developed a fear of hurting yourself, and that fear is sapping your motivation. The solution is the same. Working out with a qualified exercise therapist will help you get over this fear and start you on the road to success.

How does this apply to you? How can you relate? What are you moved to do about this issue so that you can move your body with joy?

I get bored exercising. There are many people who find "exercise" boring. So don't exercise. Find other ways to move your body. If you define exercise as going to the gym and walking on a treadmill or biking for an hour, that may not be the best form of activity for you. Perhaps walking in the park or having swimming races in the pool with your children would be more fun. Remember, you're not looking for exercise as part of a diet program so you can lose weight in the short run. You're looking for a long-term, sustainable, enjoyable form of moving your body that doesn't bore you. I would suggest you keep trying different activities, look for something new and something that maybe you wouldn't normally consider, and see if it holds your interest longer. If you love doing something, you're more likely to do it on a regular basis.

How does this apply to you? How can you relate? What are you moved to do about this issue so that you can move your body with joy?

I don't have time. In my experience, time is never the real issue. I'm sure you find time for anything you really want to do. Sometimes a lack of time as a reason not to exercise can signal the presence of an emotional block, which was the case with Carol in the story at the beginning of the chapter. We will discuss more about these emotional blocks later in this chapter. But just think of all the things you get done every single day. Ask yourself if all of them are top priority or if you can perhaps move some of them to the "if I get time" list and put physical activity higher up on your list. If you can find time to get your nails done, watch TV, and do other activities on your priority list, what would it take to make exercise a priority?

How does this apply to you? How can you relate? What are you moved to do about this issue so that you can move your body with joy?

Chapter 14: Good Eating Habits

Take Things Slowly

Eating should not be treated as a race. Eat slowly. This just means that you should take your time in relishing and enjoying your food – it's a healthy thing! So, how long do you have to grind up the food in your mouth? Well, there is no specific time food should be chewed, but 18-25 bites are enough to enjoy the food mindfully. This can be hard at first, mainly if you have been used to speed eating for a very long time. Why not try some new techniques like using chopsticks when you are accustomed to spoon and fork. Or use your non-dominant hand when eating. These strategies can slow you down and improve your awareness.

Avoid Distractions

To make things simpler for you, just make it a habit of sitting down and staying away from distractions. The handful of nuts that you eat as you walk through the kitchen and the bunch of morning snacks you nibbled while standing in front of your fridge can be hard to recall. According to researchers, people tend to eat more when they are doing other things too. You should, therefore, sit down and focus on your food to prevent mindless eating behaviors.

Savor Every Bite

Do not forget that eating mindfully is not only about enjoying the food you eat, but your health too, and without feeling guilty and uncomfortable. Relishing the sight, taste, and smell of your diet is truly worth it. This can be so easy if you take things gradually and don't rush to perfection. Make small changes towards awareness until you are a fully mindful eater. So, eat slowly and savor the good food you are eating and the proper nutrition you are giving to your body.

Surround Yourself with Positivity

Our body reacts to good vibes and bad vibes! You can easily recall the last time you were angry or upset with something, you also felt weak, dizzy and lightheaded. This is a very important thing to know that negativity impacts very badly on our body and mind. Most accidents like heart attack, stroke, high pressure, hypertension etc... all of these things occur because of reacting to negative things. On the other hand, positivity impacts very nicely to our mind and body. We feel good, we feel active, and we feel motivated to do more work. To be on a diet, you need to keep a good mood. If you are on a bad mood, you would not feel the drive to continue with the diet. You may feel skipping a day of dieting and start your cheat day on your own because you are not feeling so good. This is called emotional eating. Emotional eating is very dangerous and if you have a history of binge eating problem in the past, you must be very aware of it.

Mind the Presentation

Regardless of how busy you are; it is a good idea to set the table – making sure it looks divine. A lovely set of utensils, placement, and napkin made of eco-friendly cloth material is a perfect reminder that you need to sit down and pay attention when you have your meals.

Plate Your Food

Serving yourself and portioning your food before you bring the plate to the table can help you to consume a modest amount, rather than putting a platter on the table from which to continually replenish. You can do this even with crackers, chips, nuts and other snack foods. Keep yourself away from the temptation of eating straight from a bag of chips and different types of food. It is also helpful if you resize the bag or place the food in smaller containers so that you can stay aware of the amount of food you are eating. Having a bright idea of how much you have eaten will make you stop eating when you're full, or even sooner.

Always Choose Quality over Quantity

By making an effort to select smaller amounts of the most beautiful food within your means, you will end up enjoying and feeling satisfied without the chance of overeating. With this, it will be helpful if you spend time preparing your meals using quality and fresh ingredients. Cooking can be a pleasurable and relaxing experience if you only let yourself into it. On top of this, you can achieve the peace of mind that comes from knowing what is in the food you are eating.

Share Meals with Loved Ones

Sharing mealtime with the ones your love is a joyful thing. It may be a challenge to mix mindful eating in with your social interactions, but it is highly possible. You have to learn to pay attention both to your meal and to the conversation while eating. The two can even combine. Share your experiences regarding the textures, tastes and other elements of the food. This may feel a bit weird at first, but you will eventually have fun doing this.

Eat Slowly, with Appreciation

Sometimes they just grab something on the go and shove it down to their stomach while driving or while working. But again, you always have to make time to eat. Humans can't survive without eating. If you ever eat foods on the go and do not sit on a table to eat, you are eating mindlessly. The key to mindful eating is to sit down, eat with peace and appreciate the food in front of you. You should have time choosing what you will eat, and also time to eat it. Appreciate its taste, aroma, and texture. Think that the person who did your meal spent time doing it. They used their skills just to satisfy you.

It's important to eat slowly because it helps in better digestion, hydration, and more natural weight loss. Also, chewing your food correctly helps in better absorption. If you eat slower, you'll get the all the nutrients in the food better. And if you would start to enjoy your meal really, you could eat more mindfully. Your stress level will go down too if you eat slower.

Chew Your Food

Chewing slowly can also prevent overeating since your brain can take its time transmitting to your stomach that you are already full. When you chew properly, you eat slowly which means that you will eat lesser amount of food. You can also enjoy more of your food if you chew slowly and properly. It is when you slowdown that you develop clearer thinking. When you think clearly, you become conscious of the types of food you take in and that's when you choose the healthier one.

This is also connected to eating slowly. If you chew your diet, you will be able to eat slower. Too, chewing lets, you taste your food better. You will be surprised at all the flavors your food as if you chew it. Chewed foods are better digested, so chewing also helps in maintaining a good digestive system. The nutrients in the food will also be properly breakdown if you eat it.

To chew your food better, you could put in just small bites into your mouth. You could put a mouthful just as long as you chew it before chugging it down so that it will be better absorbed. You could chew a piece 20 to 40 times.

Take Small Bites
Eating should never be rushed. As mentioned before, you need to take your time when you eat. Sit down and feel the ambiance. Do not put everything in your mouth. You won't enjoy your food when you do that. It will also stress your digestive tract of you swallow large

bites. Your metabolism will suffer, and it could lead to weight gain. Eating should be done with pleasure, savor the taste of the food, chew thoroughly.

You could cut your food into small portions to help you take little bites. I know that it sounds easy to do, but it may be hard for those who are used to eating large meals. If you take small bits and you eat slowly, you will full sooner. It will help you eat less, but you don't get to be hungry throughout the day. You could eat another small portion when you feel hungry.

Sit Down

Eating should be done by sitting down. You should not eat while standing or while walking around because you won't enjoy your food. Also, sitting correctly makes digestion better. And you need to show some respect to your meal.

When I say sit down, it shouldn't be in front of a computer or on a park bench while you go through your cell phone. Sit down on a dining chair in your house or a restaurant or any place suitable for decent dining. If you are multitasking, you would have a hard time appreciating what you are eating. You will tend to eat fast, and you won't have time to chew and break down your food. Stop eating on the go. If you want to lead a healthy life, just do it now.

Pick the Smaller Plate

You might think that the size of the plate does not matter, but it does. If you have large dishes at home, it is the time that you change them to something smaller. We tend to put food that will cover the space on the plate, and we think that it's enough amount. Also if you see less, you might crave less. Using smaller plate is vital for portion control.

Start by changing the plates at your house. If you are a buffet lover, then it's better if you pick up smaller dishes instead of the big ones. It will help you control the amount of food you will put on the plate.

Chapter 15: Meditation for Eating Well

When you think of meditation, you might picture a serene place with little or no distraction, providing an opportunity to let your stress, thoughts, and judgments slide away for a deep sense of relaxation. This is ideal, though isn't the reality for most of our time, which is spent keeping busy, going from one task to the next, with little or no time for rest in between. Meditation, however, can be practiced anywhere once you can become accustomed to tuning out distractions and focus on your thoughts and feelings. This is crucial and the basis for successful intuitive eating.

Envision positivity, as the first step to intuitive eating. Think about your goals, whether they are weight loss, better health, improving your energy, food choices, and overall well-being. This will provide a focus on what you want to achieve. Meditation begins with letting go of all the negativity and judgments we make about ourselves, our food and body image. Dedicate time, as little or as much as you can, to "checking in" with your body and mind, at least once a day. This will take time to get accustomed to, though it will become easier with practice. Only ten minutes each day is the session is needed, though more time can be added as it becomes available. There are some points to remember as you incorporate mindful meditation into your daily schedule.

Stay positive. Keep your thoughts positive. Instead of criticizing or judging your actions, appearance or habits, try to find the positive. Take note of how inner criticisms impact you. Each time you chastise yourself for a mistake, note how you feel: do your shoulders tense up or stomach tighten? As soon as you realize this reaction, it will become easier to release the tension: lower your shoulders, take deep breaths and focus on something you accomplished, anything at all that brings a sense of confidence. This could be something as simple as finishing an errand successfully, meeting a deadline, or just acknowledging your need for self-care, which is a good move in itself! Avoid telling yourself that you need to lose weight, that you are not worthy or good enough. We constantly place a lot of pressure on ourselves to meet deadlines, goals and are subject to a lot in our daily lives. Take the time to break away and give yourself that positive boost and recognize that daily need for self-care.

Change your environment. This is a challenge if you have a hectic family life or work schedule. There are some opportunities to find space within these constraints: early morning or before bed. The first step is to calm your surroundings with less distraction and noise. This can be accomplished by wearing a pair of sleep headphones that block out background sounds. Another option is to play soothing ocean waves, rain and various nature backgrounds to transport your mind to a peaceful zone. This will set your mind in a serene state where you can envision yourself in a calm place, where negativity, compulsions to make hasty decisions, including food cravings, melt away. If you choose to listen to guided meditation recordings or practice self-hypnosis, this can be done in the same way. Take the time to find a quiet corner in your home or office and start practicing this once a day for ten or fifteen minutes.

Reward your busy lifestyle with non-food rewards. Cravings for food often occur when we face emotional situations that cause us stress. We may also experience them during happier moments when we dine with friends or family and feel a sense of compulsion. It takes only a snap decision to make a choice to satisfy the craving or become mindful at the moment and divert our attention from it. Food is often used as a reward system. "Have the cake; you deserve it!" There is nothing wrong with having a cake or a treat; it's the reason behind it. Food can become a system to feed our feelings and sense of need, even when we aren't hungry. One way to change this pattern is to reward ourselves with non-food items. For example, if you have an argument or disagreement or a stressful day, draw yourself a warm bath. Add Epsom salts, essential oils and scents that you find calming. Lavender, rosemary, sage are good choices for a soothing experience.

Treat yourself to a home spa, or if you can, visit a salon, museum or art gallery to pause all the motion in your life and focus on beauty, history and the arts. This can help aid you with meditation and self-reflection, as you notice the effects these activities have on you. If you have other interests, such as sports and nature, a bicycle ride or getting involved in a group sport can be a great distraction from food, either individually or with a team. Arts and crafts provide another way to focus your attention on creating a reward, and studies have shown positive effects on the body and mind. There are many other activities that can provide a new way to calm and reward your mind and body for all that you do.

Gentle exercise for gentle nutrition. As with intuitive eating's gentle approach to nutrition, exercise can be approached in a similar way. Binge eating and exercise are two extreme issues that plague dieters. When you overeat or binge outside of a diet plan, one reaction may be to over-exercise to compensate for the additional calories and carbohydrates consumed. In effect, it can be seen as a form of self-punishment to "correct" this action. With a more balanced view of eating and exercise, this is never required and should be avoided.

If you engage in high impact sports, such as martial arts, weightlifting, cycling and HIIT (high impact interval training), you'll notice benefits from these activities, though more moderate movement options are available to you if these options are not realistic. Walking is a good moderate form of exercise for people who are unable to participate in more vigorous sports. Swimming and aqua-fit classes are a good option for people with limited mobility due to joint pain and chronic conditions that impact movement. Yoga and gentle stretching can achieve a lot of flexibility and mindfulness at the same time. Choose an exercise that fits best within your life and abilities, as all forms of movement provide a positive impact on your mind and body.

Mindful exercise for a good night's rest. Our eating habits are shaped by how well we rest. If we oversleep or do not get enough rest, this can impact our cravings and sense of needing more food to function better, even if we are not hungry. The most common example is a craving for sugar or caffeine, both of which can be very addictive and are consumed in large amounts on a daily basis. Coffee is one of the most consumed beverages in the world, surpassing alcohol and other popular drinks. A busy schedule and hectic life can also mess with our sleeping patterns. There is a way to meditate or prepare for sleep in a way that is beneficial for your mind and eating habits by following these steps:

1.Find a comfortable space to lie down or sit, preferably on a firm, yet soft surface to allow your body to relax

2.Take a deep breath. Count as you inhale, from one to five, then hold the breath in, counting to five again, then slowly exhale, at the same pace, for five. Repeat this with your eyes closed or half closed, whichever is most calming.

3.Visualize your breath as a wave, coming in and out, and taking with it all negative thoughts and emotions. Creating this visual in our mind will help dissolve the stress we carry inside, resulting in the sense of relief

4.Clear your thoughts and focus on the present. We are so accustomed to doing and thinking, instead of just being.

Scan your body from head to feet. This is a practice that mentally processes each part or section of your body to note any signs of tightness, tension, soreness or stress:

1.Begin with your head, neck, and shoulders. Do you feel any ache or tension? Often, we hold our shoulders up towards our ears, even in a state of relaxation or rest. Once we notice this, we can let them fall away, down towards the ground, opening the area around our ears.

2.Traveling down towards our chest, do you notice any shallow breathing? When we inhale, does the air come from our chest, stomach or diaphragm? If you are experiencing an upset stomach, take some deep breaths, counting to five with each inhales and exhales, keeping it even.

3.Scan both arms, further down your chest and the rest of your body, noting any areas of muscle pain, tension or sensitivity. As you come across areas of concern, take deep breaths and focus your energy in these spots. This will make you mindful of which areas need more care and attention.

Calm foods and drink before bed. Bedtime snacks are often discouraged and for a good reason: they may not be digested as well and may interfere with your sleep. This doesn't mean you have to avoid them completely. An herbal tea, a small piece of fruit can be an effective way to satisfy mild hunger and help you to relax before bed. The fruit is light and can be digested within thirty minutes, which is quicker than other foods, leaving you satisfied, though not overfed before bed.

Herbal teas, such as chamomile, or mint, can have a soothing effect on your body, preparing you for sleep.

If you prefer a piece of fruit, a banana, a small cup of berries or piece of melon is a good light snack, half an hour before bedtime. Another option is yogurt, which contains probiotics and can rest a sensitive stomach.

Daily affirmations and positivity in everyday life. We are bombarded with demands and high expectations. Take a moment every day to congratulate yourself on doing all that you can and appreciate yourself for who you are and what you have in your life. This is an exercise that can be done every morning, in the bathroom, bedroom or outside, if that is an available option. Take a few minutes to give yourself self-love and the pat on the back for all that you accomplish. Speak out loud if you can, to hear these positive words in your own voice. Write them down and post them in a familiar place:

I can accomplish what I put my mind to.

I'm capable of doing good and achieving things.

I will succeed.

If this day is difficult, I can handle it, and the next will be better.

If I encounter a challenge, I will face and conquer it.

There are many positive phrases and affirmations that can be found online, in books and that you can make on your own. Use these to start your day with a fresh, renewed outlook on life, where you control your own destiny and achieve your goals.

Conclusion

I know some of what I have said so far may seem a little conflicting. After all how can you love yourself and do what pleases you, when what pleases you is eating like ten bowls of chocolate ice cream and yet maintain a healthy food balance?

I never said it was going to be easy. I am just suggesting you mix a bit of confidence and self-love with a healthy diet. You will be wowed by the results.

Our emotions are very powerful. If we can manage to use positive energy to influence our emotions, we will have really good feelings. Have you ever been around someone at work that seems to always be happy, smiling, talking to people, laughing at every single thing, and you wonder if they ever for any reason feel angry or sad? Well, these people just know how to channel more positive energy.

It's that simple!
Give yourself a reason to laugh or smile. If people don't do it for you, find joy in the little things around you. Spend your time positively. I am sure we all know an idle mind is said to be the devil's workshop! Do not

spend idle time contemplating what to eat. Instead, spend it on worthwhile ventures. Everybody has something they have always wanted to do. What's it for you?

It's so easy to blame other people or things for how we are feeling, but people refuse to accept that they are responsible for their emotions. If something makes you mad, talk about it to someone. If you can't, gear up, go to the gym with the picture of the person who made you mad, imagine giving them much needed lessons on boxing.

Find an outlet!

Emotional eating in a lot of people is born from repressed emotions. Some people feel crying makes them look weak. Others feel like calling people out on their crap might hurt the person's feelings. So does this mean it's okay for you to be hurt and just suffer in silence? *No way!*

Go on up to that person and say, "Hey you, I do not like what you said. Kindly offer an apology." If they won't give it, learn to accept that and be okay without it. If you know you were also in the wrong, apologize first. That way, they are more likely to tender an honest apology, and when they do? Forgive them and move on.

Forgiveness is not for them. It's for you! It's just a fancy name for unshackling yourself from a particular issue.

Whatever you're going through, be proactive about finding joy, whether you recently suffered a breakup, you just lost your job or a loved one, someone called you Fatty NcFatterson... It' doesn't matter! Know you are perfect. You deserve to be loved. You especially deserve love from *you.* I'm willing to bet there is someone out there who is dying to meet you! He or she is probably praying every night to have you in their lives. You just haven't met them yet. So, put yourself out there, interact, socialize and you might just get a step closer to meeting your better half.

Ah! The smell of potential love is in the air!
You need emotions to survive. Don't try to suppress them. Find healthy ways to express them. Let them out and let them go. Don't bury it all deep down inside till you start feeling emotional hunger again.

Take the wheel of your life, and drive! Drive responsibly. Imagine your emotions are a new Bugatti you just bought. Of course you would drive carefully and avoid leaving scratches on your new baby!

Handle your emotions with just as much attention and care!
Nurture them, direct them, take care of them, and do not let them get you into trouble. Because unruly emotions bring about emotional eating, along with health complications and other eating disorders.

Love Yourself

You have to learn to love yourself so others can love you. It doesn't matter if you have a good sized stomach or a generous behind. There is this aura confident people who love themselves give off.

Have you ever walked beside someone and thought to yourself this person feels good about themselves? We usually think that because this person walks ramrod straight with a pep in their step and the wind in their hair. It's not just what you are seeing. It's what they believe about themselves that you see and feel! That's the energy they are giving off, and you just can't help but really sense it. If you look closely, you might see a zit or two, even a mole somewhere. But it doesn't matter because that self-love and confidence they exude just blinds you to all that. So be that guy!

Feel good about yourself! If only you knew how many people in the world want to be like you. Someone somewhere is tired of being too skinny or too short or tall, while you want to be as skinny or as whatever as they are. It's human nature to want what we can't or don't have. It's even taught in economics that humans are insatiable. You might wish you were skinny now, but if you actually were, you would understand the struggles of a skinny person. Appreciate what you have now because someone somewhere wants it.

Everyone Is Unique

We are all unique beings. Our genes and environment play a huge role in how we look. You can't come from a family of generously proportioned people and expect to be as thin as a reed. Not without doing some work! Accept what you are, and do what you can to change it to what you prefer. You don't have to loathe yourself along the way to change.

Emotional eating is an issue. A big one.

if you feel you are an emotional eater but you aren't really sure, talk to someone who listens and might understand. If you are for any reason too shy for that, you could dedicate a little of time to research. Try to check what level of seriousness yours has gotten to. If it is quite serious, try to see an expert. Do not do anything drastic.

We all have problems. We have things that may keep wide awake late into the night; things that cause us to worry, fear, or push us to anger. It's how we deal with these things that matter.

For example, you may have lost your job. See it as a new opportunity to further your career.

Did you really mean to work for someone else for the rest of your life, anyway? There are many opportunities out there. You could come up with something new, or if you can't, follow one of the many job trends out there. Just try to be a bit innovative. Who knows, you might be the change we have all been looking forward to!

Be Easy About This

The problem is we try to conform to a certain structure. We are all afraid of exploring and trying new things, because we are afraid to fail.

Well, you won't know until you try! So try!
So what if you fall flat on your face when you begin working on your emotional eating issues? Pick yourself up and start again. Just because you stepped out of

line once or twice in a row doesn't mean you should call it quits. Stop being so hard on yourself!

Explore The New

Do you love to dance but really don't know how? Why not go for dancing lessons then? It's a form of exercise and it helps keep your mind occupied.

Travel somewhere else and learn about their culture and practices. It's never too late to learn something new! You don't always have to limit your travels to the images in a travel book.

Deal With It

The best way of dealing with situations is to meet them head on. Try strategic methods of approach. Or, if you know they are not important at all and unnecessarily bothering you, then forget it! Some problems just come to challenge your resolve. You don't have to let that one thing win. Don't let it drag you under and push you into unhealthy habits.

Live! Love! Learn!

Every waking moment is a learning experience, so be open to new opportunities. Be a willing student of life. There is no limit to learning. When you are engaged in productive activities, time seems to fly by in a blur. You won't even have time for unhealthy eating habits.

As long as you live, there are better options and opportunities out there. You haven't even tried one-third of them yet, so how can you claim to be bored? Have you read every novel, magazine or comic there is? Or listened to every song ever sung? Or participated in every game known to man?

You, my dear, have no excuse.
The only thing you can do for yourself is to live a good, and healthy life. You will be grateful for it in your old age.

So, grab opportunities and live the best life you can.

Made in the USA
Coppell, TX
21 June 2020